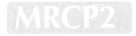

Practice Questions & Answers

HIV and Genitourinary Medicine and Infectious Diseases

 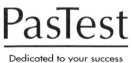

PasTest

Dedicated to your success

MRCP2

Practice Questions & Answers

HIV and Genitourinary Medicine and Infectious Diseases

Edited by

Philip Kelly MBBS MRCP

Department of Endocrinology

St Bartholomew's Hospital

Barts and The London NHS Trust

London

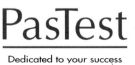

Dedicated to your success

© 2006 PASTEST LTD
Egerton Court
Parkgate Estate
Knutsford
Cheshire
WA16 8DX

Telephone: 01565 752000

First Published 2006

ISBN: 1 904627 870

A catalogue record for this book is available from the British Library.

The information contained within this book was obtained by the author from reliable
sources. However, while every effort has been made to ensure its accuracy, no
responsibility for loss, damage or injury occasioned to any person acting or refraining
from action as a result of information contained herein can be accepted by the
publishers or author.

PasTest Revision Books and Intensive Courses
PasTest has been established in the field of postgraduate medical education since
1972, providing revision books and intensive study courses for doctors preparing for
their professional examinations. Books and courses are available for the following
specialties:
**MRCGP, MRCP Parts 1 and 2, MRCPCH Parts 1 and 2, MRCPsych, MRCS,
MRCOG Parts 1 and 2, DRCOG, DCH, FRCA,
PLAB Parts 1 and 2.**

For further details contact:
**PasTest, Freepost, Knutsford, Cheshire WA16 7BR
Tel: 01565 752000   Fax: 01565 650264
Email: enquiries@pastest.co.uk   Web site: www.pastest.co.uk**

Text prepared by Vision Typesetting, Manchester
Printed and bound in the UK by the Alden Group, Oxfordshire

CONTENTS

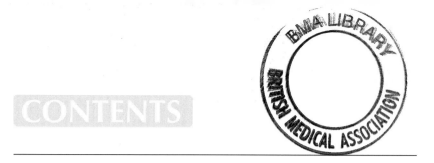

CONTRIBUTORS

Benjamin M Clark MBChB MRCP DTM&H
Specialist Registrar in Infectious Diseases
Department of Infection and Tropical Medicine
Royal Hallamshire Hospital, Sheffield, UK

Mun-Yee Tung MBBS MRCP
Specialist Registrar in Genitourinary Medicine
Chelsea and Westminster Hospital, London, UK

ACKNOWLEDGEMENTS

I would like to express my gratitude to the team at PasTest particularly to Amy Smith and Cathy Dickens for their patience and support during the preparation of this volume. Many patients have been gracious enough to contribute to our ongoing education by allowing their images to be used in this volume. Thanks are due to Dr Alexandra Nanzer who provided assistance with the proof reading.

Ben Clark would like to thank the following colleagues and institutions for their help in the preparation of his questions:
Tim Clarke, MLSO2, Department of Microbiology, Royal Hallamshire Hospital, Sheffield, UK
Dr Charles Romanowski, Consultant Neuroradiologist, Royal Hallamshire Hospital, Sheffield, UK
Dr Parminder Chaggar, Senior House Officer, Royal Hallamshire Hospital, Sheffield, UK
Dr Claire Dewsnap, Specialist Registrar, Genito-Urinary Medicine Department, Royal Hallamshire Hospital, Sheffield, UK
Agricultural Research Service Photo Unit, United States Department of Agriculture

Philip Kelly

Picture Permissions

Image page 61 (From Wheat, LJ *et al*. Pulmonary Histoplasmosis Syndromes: Recognition, Diagnosis and Management. *Seminars in Respiratory and Critical Care Medicine* 2004; 25: 129–145. Reprinted by permission.)

INTRODUCTION

The MRCP (UK) Part 2 written examination consists of three 3-hour papers, each with up to 100 multiple choice questions; they are either one from five (best of five) or 'n' from many, where any number of answers are chosen from ten options. Each question will have a clinical scenario and might contain investigations to interpret; many might also contain an image. There is a pass mark agreed by the examiners but a candidate's performance is also assessed in relation to other candidates. This book contains practice questions written by current registrars in both infectious diseases and HIV and genitourinary medicine. They are experienced enough in supervising their own, and other juniors to know where the 'gaps' in the knowledge are – alongside their own successful recent passage through the MRCP examinations, and hence these questions are essential aids to preparation for the examination.

The authors have been chosen for their clear understanding of their topics and how they relate to the uncertain world of not only the MRCP but also when receiving and reviewing patients on the wards, in the emergency department or in clinic. As such, this title is not only useful to those sitting the MRCP; it will also be of use to consultants and registrars wanting to brush up their skills for the general take and house officers and medical students wanting a more thorough understanding of the complex diagnostic and management problems one can be faced with. The breadth of knowledge required for the exam is vast and the authors have attempted to cover the 'syllabus' as completely as possible. Great care has been taken to explain areas of difficulty as thoroughly as possible. No apology is made where the format of the questions differs slightly from the exam. These books are not merely practice papers but educational aids, where a topic can best be explained by diversion from the strict format of the exam, for the sake of understanding, this has been done.

This book is best taken – in concert with the first three books in the series – as a supplement to a thorough clinical grounding, the general medical texts and the core clinical journals.

Any comments and suggestions on this book or the series will be gratefully received.

α-FP	α-fetoprotein
A&E	Accident & Emergency department
AAFB	Acid-alcohol fast bacteria
ABG	Arterial blood gases
ABPA	Allergic bronchopulmonary aspergillosis
ACE	Angiotensin-converting enzyme
ADH	Antidiuretic hormone
AFB	Acid-fast bacteria
ALA	Amoebic liver abscess
ALP	Alkaline phosphatase
AMTS	Abbreviated mini-mental test score
ANA	Antinuclear antibody
ANCA	Anti-neutrophil cytoplasmic antibody
AP	Anteroposterior
APC	Activated protein C
APTT	Activated partial thromboplastin time
ARDS	Acute respiratory distress syndrome
AST	Aspartate aminotransferase
AXR	Abdominal X-ray
BAL	bronchoalveolar lavage fluid
BCG	Bacillus Calmette-Guérin
BMT	Bone marrow transplant
bpm	beats per minute
cAb	Core antibody
CCHF	Congo-Crimean haemorrhagic fever
CFT	Complement fixation test
CK	Creatine kinase
CLO	Campylobacter like organism – the test for *Helicobacter pylori*
CMV	Cytomegalovirus
CNS	Central nervous system

COPD	Chronic obstructive pulmonary disease
CRAG	Cryptococcal antigen test
CRP	C-reactive protein
CSF	Cerebrospinal fluid
CT	Computed tomography
CXR	Chest X-ray
D+V	Diarrhoea and vomiting
DEAFF	Detection of Early Antigen Fluorescent Foci
DEET	N, N-Diethyl-meta-Toluamide (insect repellent)
DIC	Disseminated intravascular coagulation
DOT	Directly observed therapy
EBNA	Epstein-Barr nuclear antigen
EBV	Epstein-Barr virus
ECG	Electrocardiogram
EEG	Electroencephalogram
EIA	Enzyme immunoassay
ELISA	Enzyme-linked immunoassay
ESR	Erythrocyte sedimentation rate
FBC	Full blood count
FDA	Food and Drug Adminstration
FSGS	Focal segmental glomerulosclerosis
FTA	Fluorescent treponemal antibody
GBM	Glomerular basement membrane
GCS	Glasgow Coma Scale
G-CSF	Granulocyte colony-stimulating factor
GI	Gastrointestinal
GM-CSF	Granulocyte-macrophage colony-stimulating factor
GN	Glomerulonephritis
GP	General practitioner
GVHD	Graft-versus-host disease
HAART	Highly active anti-retroviral therapy
Hb	Haemoglobin
HCC	Hepatocellular carcinoma
HCG	Human chorionic gonadotrophin
HCV	Hepatitis C virus
HCW	Health-care worker
HHV-1	Human herpesvirus 1
HiB	*Haemophilus influenzae* type B
HIV	Human immunodeficiency virus
HIV-AN	Human immunodeficiency virus-associated nephropathy

HLA	Human leukocyte antigen
HPA	Health Protection Agency
HRCT	High-resolution computed tomography
HSV-1	Herpes simplex virus 1
HTLV-1	Human T-cell leukaemia virus 1
HUS	Haemolytic-uraemic syndrome
IFAT	Immunofluorescent antibody testing
IgG	Immunoglobulin G
ITU	Intensive Therapy Unit
IUCD	Intrauterine contraceptive device
iv	intravenous
JVP	Jugular venous pulse/pressure
KS	Kaposi's sarcoma
LDH	Lactate dehydrogenase
LFT	Liver function test
MAT	Microscopic agglutination test
MCV	Mean corpuscular volume
MDRTB	Multi-drug-resistant tuberculosis
MRCP	Magnetic resonance cholangiopancreatography
MRI	Magnetic resonance imaging
MRSA	Methycillin-resistant *Staphylococcus aureus*
NNN	Novy, MacNeal, Nicolle media
NSAID	Non-steroidal anti-inflammatory drug
OGD	Oesophago-gastro-duodenoscopy
PAS	Periodic Acid Schiff
PCP	**P**neumo*cystis jiroveci* **p**neumonia – formerly known as **P**neumo*cystis* **c**arinii **p**neumonia
PCR	Polymerase chain reaction
PEG-IFN	Polyethylene glycol-interferon
PEP	Post-exposure prophylaxis
PLA	Pyogenic liver abscess
PT	Prothrombin time
RBC	Red blood cell
RF	Rheumatoid factor
RIA	Radioimmunoassay
RPR	Rapid Plasma Reagin

sAb	Surface antibody
sAg	Surface antigen
SARS	Severe Acute Respiratory Syndrome
SEB	Staphylococcal enterotoxin B
SIADH	Syndrome of inappropriate ADH secretion
SVR	Sustained viral response
TB	Tuberculosis
TBM	Tuberculous meningitis
TPHA	*Treponema pallidum* haemagglutination test
TPPA	*Treponema pallidum* particle agglutination
TSS	Toxic shock syndrome
TSST-1	Toxic shock syndrome toxin 1
TTE	Transthoracic echocardiogram
TTP	Thrombotic thrombocytopenic purpura
U&E	Urea and electrolytes
US	Ultrasound
UTI	Urinary tract infection
VCA	Viral capsid antigen
VDRL	Veneral Diseases Research Laboratory
WCC	White cell count
WHO	World Health Organization
WHO/IUATLD	WHO/International Union Against Tuberculosis and Lung Disease

Chapter One

HIV AND GENITOURINARY MEDICINE

Case 1

A 32-year-old man presents to A&E with a 1-month history of a non-productive cough, loss of appetite, and fever. He has had neither chest pain nor orthopnoea. He previously had asthma; his current medication consists of salbutamol and beclomethasone inhalers. Ten days earlier he had been to see his GP who prescribed him a week's course of amoxicillin 500 mg tds with no improvement.

On examination he is breathless with a temperature of 38.5°C, with oxygen saturations of 92% on room air. He has cervical lymphadenopathy and on auscultation there are bilateral basal crepitations.

Investigations:

Hb	10.7 g/dL
WCC	4.2×10^9/L
Neutrophils	3.5×10^9/L
Platelets	92×10^9/L
Sodium	138 mmol/L
Potassium	4.2 mmol/L
Urea	7.0 mmol/L
Creatinine	95 µmol/L
Bilirubin	10 µmol/L
AST	40 U/L
ALP	120 U/L
Albumin	28 U/L
CRP	22 mg/L

Arterial Blood Gas (ABG) – on room air

pH	7.32
P_{CO_2}	4.6 kPa
P_{O_2}	7.8 kPa
Bicarbonate	17 mmol/L

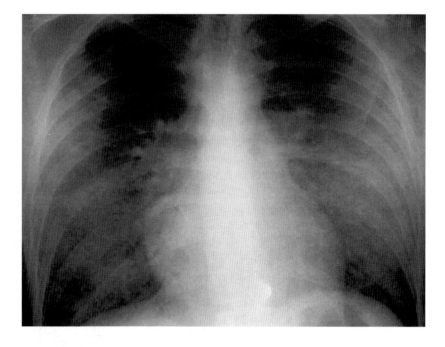

1 Which is the most likely diagnosis?

- A *Streptococcus pneumoniae* pneumonia
- B Pulmonary tuberculosis (TB)
- C *Pneumocystis carinii* pneumonia
- D Poorly controlled asthma
- E Sarcoidosis

2 What two tests would help you confirm the diagnosis?

- A Blood cultures
- B Serial arterial blood gases
- C Exercise oximetry
- D Mycoplasma serology
- E TB blood cultures
- F Mantoux test
- G Induced sputum
- H Lung function tests
- I Acute and convalescent atypical serology
- J Open lung biopsy

Case 2

A 38-year-old gay man presents with a rash on his skin. He has no other symptoms.

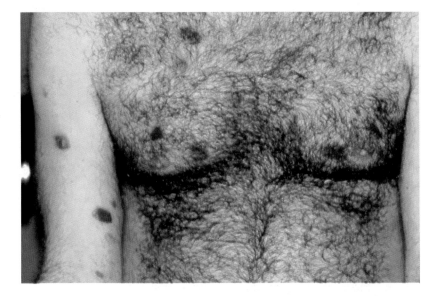

1   Which is the most likely diagnosis?

- [ ] A   Bacillary angiomatosis
- [ ] B   Haematomas secondary to thrombocytopenia
- [ ] C   Fixed drug eruption
- [ ] D   Kaposi's sarcoma
- [ ] E   Pyogenic granulomas

2   What is the causative agent?

- [ ] A   *Bartonella henselae*
- [ ] B   Human herpes virus 8
- [ ] C   Epstein–Barr virus
- [ ] D   *Mycobacterium tuberculosis*
- [ ] E   Human immunodeficiency virus

Case 3

A 27-year-old man presents to clinic with a 4-week history of a rash on the soles of his feet and pain in his ankles. Six weeks previously he had been treated with ciprofloxacin for an acute diarrhoeal illness.

On examination:

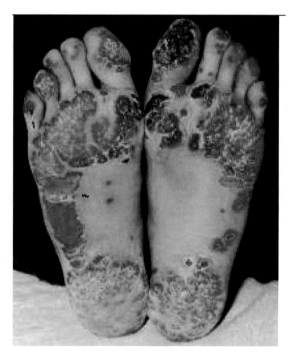

1 Which is the most likely diagnosis?

- ☐ A Stevens–Johnson syndrome
- ☐ B Parvovirus B19 infection
- ☐ C Fixed drug eruption
- ☐ D Secondary syphilis
- ☐ E Keratoderma blennorrhagica

2 What is the causative agent?

- ☐ A Ciprofloxacin
- ☐ B Parvovirus B19
- ☐ C Salmonella
- ☐ D Herpes simplex virus
- ☐ E *Treponema pallidum*

Case 4

A 42-year-old man presents with a 4-day history of fever, nausea, vomiting, and lower abdominal pain. There is no past medical history of note. He lives with his partner of 3 years. He takes no medication. He has no known allergies.

On examination the temperature is 38°C. There is a faint maculopapular rash on his trunk. Abdominal examination elicits suprapubic tenderness and a tender right hypochondrium. Rectal examination is normal as is urinalysis.

Investigations are as follows:

Hb	12.3 g/dL
WCC	2.2×10^9/L
Neutrophils	1.6×10^9/L
Platelets	80×10^9/L
Sodium	135 mmol/L
Potassium	4.5 mmol/L
Urea	4.6 mmol/L
Creatinine	78 µmol/L
Bilirubin	15 µmol/L
AST	30 U/L
ALP	130 U/L
Albumin	30 U/L
CRP	12 mg/L
Hepatitis B sAg	negative
Hepatitis B cAb	negative
Hepatitis C Ab	negative
Hepatitis A IgM	negative
HIV 1+2 Ab	negative

1   Which is the best test to confirm diagnosis?

☐   A   Hepatitis C genotype
☐   B   P24 antigen
☐   C   Repeat HIV antibody test using a different testing kit
☐   D   HIV viral load
☐   E   EBV serology

Case 5

A 45-year-old man has been recently diagnosed HIV positive. He discloses a 3-month history of watery diarrhoea with weight loss. He has had no recent foreign travel.

On examination the temperature is 37.8°C, he looks thin and has oropharyngeal candidiasis. Blood pressure 125/80 mmHg, the chest is clear, and in the abdomen no abnormality is detected. There is no focal neurology.

Investigations:

Hb	10.8 g/dL
WCC	4.2 × 10⁹/L
Neutrophils	2.8 × 10⁹/L
Platelets	110 × 10⁹/L
Sodium	144 mmol/L
Potassium	4.3 mmol/L
Urea	4.5 mmol/L
Creatinine	70 µmol/L
Bilirubin	7 µmol/L
AST	20 U/L
ALP	90 U/L
Albumin	28 U/L
CRP	7 mg/L
CD4 count	90 cells/mm³
Viral load	95,000 copies/mL

Stool	
M, C & S	negative
Ova, cysts, parasites	oocysts of cryptosporidium

1   What is the best treatment to commence?

☐ A   Metronidazole
☐ B   Metronidazole + combination antiretroviral therapy
☐ C   Ciprofloxacin + combination antiretroviral therapy
☐ D   Fluconazole
☐ E   Combination antiretroviral therapy

Case 6

A 42-year-old man with long-standing HIV infection for 9 years is admitted for investigation of an 8-week history of weight loss, diarrhoea, pain on defecation, and abdominal pain. He has never taken antiretroviral therapy.

On observation: he is very thin and cachectic, the temperature is 38.2°C, blood pressure 110/70 mmHg. The chest is clear. Abdominal examination elicits right upper quadrant tenderness and there is no peritonism. Fundoscopy reveals a small area of perivascular infiltrate with haemorrhage near the macula. There is no focal neurology.

Investigations:

Hb	10.3 g/dL
WCC	5.0×10^9/L
Neutrophils	3.8×10^9/L
Platelets	100×10^9/L
Sodium	140 mmol/L
Potassium	4.5 mmol/L
Urea	5.5 mmol/L
Creatinine	60 µmol/L
Bilirubin	10 µmol/L
AST	30 U/L
ALP	700 U/L
Albumin	29 U/L
CRP	3 mg/L
CD_4 count	29 cells/mm³
Viral load	120,000 copies/mL

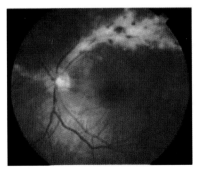

1   What is the best treatment to commence?

☐ A   Aciclovir iv
☐ B   Septrin iv
☐ C   Amphotericin iv
☐ D   Ganciclovir iv
☐ E   Combination antiretroviral therapy

2   What test do you order to investigate his abdominal symptoms?

☐ A   Colonoscopy
☐ B   CT abdomen with contrast
☐ C   Liver biopsy
☐ D   Gastroscopy
☐ E   Laporoscopy

Case 7

A 42-year-old woman presents with a 5-day history of fever and headache, and a 1-day history of confusion. She is a former intravenous drug user and she was diagnosed HIV and hepatitis C positive 9 months ago. Her baseline CD4 count was 192 cells/mm³ with a viral load of 32,000 copies/mL. She defaulted from follow-up until this presentation.

On examination the temperature is 38.1°C, heart rate 100 bpm, blood pressure 95/50 mmHg, the chest is clear; CNS – GCS 14/15, photophobia, neck stiffness, no rash, and no focal neurology.

Investigations:

Hb	8.8 g/dL
WCC	3.0×10^9/L
Neutrophils	2.5×10^9/L
Platelets	90×10^9/L
Sodium	135 mmol/L
Potassium	3.5 mmol/L
Urea	7.5 mmol/L
Creatinine	80 μmol/L
Bilirubin	7 μmol/L
AST	22 U/L
ALP	100 U/L
Albumin	27 U/L

CD4 count	13 cells/mm³
Viral load	>500,000 copies/mL

CT brain with contrast – no focal lesions, no evidence of raised intracranial pressure

Lumbar puncture – opening pressure 35 cmH$_2$O
CSF microscopy – RBC <1, WCC 10, no organism seen on Gram stain

CSF glucose	0.8 mmol/L
CSF protein	3.2 g/L

1 What investigation will confirm the diagnosis?

- [ ] A CSF India ink stain
- [ ] B CSF VDRL
- [ ] C CSF PCR
- [ ] D CSF silver stain
- [ ] E CSF Ziehl–Neelsen stain

11

Case 8

A 62-year-old man is referred with progressive confusion, ataxia, and decreased mobility and with a 1-day history of seizures. His past medical history is that he was recently diagnosed as HIV-positive and his last CD4 count was 92 cells/mm³ with a viral load of 77,000 copies/mL. He had just started antiretroviral therapy 3 weeks ago. He has had no previous strokes, has no history of ischaemic heart disease, and is not diabetic.

On examination: temperature is 38.1°C, heart rate 100 bpm, blood pressure 95/50 mmHg, the chest is clear, the abdomen reveals no palpable organs; in the CNS the GCS is 14/15, there is no photophobia, neck stiffness or rash. He is drowsy and confused with no localising signs elicited.

An urgent brain CT scan demonstrated six ring-enhancing mass lesions in the left postero-temporal area and the basal ganglia with surrounding oedema.

1   What treatment should you prescribe?

- [ ] A   Rifampicin, isoniazid, pyrazinamide, and ethambutol
- [ ] B   Sulphadiazine and pyrimethamine
- [ ] C   Amphotericin B
- [ ] D   Ceftriaxone and vancomycin
- [ ] E   Cranial irradiation + cisplatin chemotherapy

Case 9

A 29-year-old man is newly diagnosed HIV positive. He is a gay man and his regular male partner has also just been diagnosed. He presents to clinic for the first time since being diagnosed to get his blood results.

Investigations:

CD4 count	22 cells/mm^3
Viral load	70,000 copies/mL
Hepatitis B sAg	negative
Hepatitis B cAb	negative
Hepatitis B sAb	negative
Hepatitis C Ab	negative
Hepatitis A IgG	positive

1   Which other medication should you commence as prophylaxis for opportunistic infection apart from co-trimoxazole?

☐ A   Doxycycline
☐ B   Azithromycin
☐ C   Amoxicillin
☐ D   Ciprofloxacin
☐ E   Nystatin

2   Which vaccination would you not be recommending?

☐ A   Influenza
☐ B   Hepatitis B
☐ C   Tetanus
☐ D   BCG
☐ E   Pneumococcal vaccine

Case 10

A 26-year-old lady from Zimbabwe is diagnosed HIV-positive through routine antenatal testing at 24 weeks gestation. This is her first pregnancy. She is asymptomatic. Anomaly scan reveals a healthy singleton fetus with no anomalies detected. She has no known allergies.

Investigations:

CD4 count	312 cells/mm^3
Viral load	70,000 copies/mL
Hepatitis B sAg	negative
Hepatitis B cAb	negative
Hepatitis B sAb	negative
Hepatitis C Ab	negative
Rubella IgG	positive
VDRL	1 : 128
TPPA	positive
FTA	positive

1   Which is the best treatment for her?

- [ ] A   Benzathine penicillin
- [ ] B   Procaine penicillin
- [ ] C   Amoxicillin
- [ ] D   Doxycycline
- [ ] E   Erythromycin

Case 11

A nurse sustains a needle-stick injury following venepuncture of a patient, known to be a current injecting drug user. You are asked to assess her on the ward.

The most recent available serological results of the donor patient are from 2 years earlier.

Hepatitis B cAb	positive
Hepatitis B sAg	negative
Hepatitis C antibody	positive
Hepatitis C PCR	negative
HIV antibody	negative

1 Which one of the following is true?

☐ A The risk of HIV transmission following a needle-stick injury from an HIV-positive patient is approximately 1–2%

☐ B Regardless of her hepatitis B immune status the nurse should be given hepatitis B immunoglobulin (HBIG)

☐ C She should be offered post-exposure prophylaxis for HIV infection

☐ D The risk of hepatitis C infection in this case is negligible

☐ E The source patient does not need to give consent before further serological blood tests are performed on his blood samples

Case 12

A 72-year-old man presents with several months of increasing confusion. He was born in Jamaica and moved to the UK in the 1960s with his current wife.

The only abnormalities in his blood tests are:

TPPA	positive
VDRL	negative
Treponemal EIA IgM	negative
Treponemal EIA IgG	positive

1   Which one of the following is not true?

- A   The results are consistent with late latent syphilis
- B   The results are consistent with secondary syphilis
- C   The results are consistent with previously treated syphilis
- D   The results are consistent with non-venereal treponemal infection
- E   His wife needs treponemal serology performing

Chapter Two

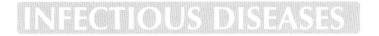

Case 1

A 29-year-old doctor develops a rash on her arms and legs. It is painful and associated with general malaise and an intermittent low-grade fever. She arrived in the UK 2 years ago after having previously lived and worked in India. There is no past medical history and she is on no regular medication.

On examination she has the rash shown below. There is nothing else of note on examination.

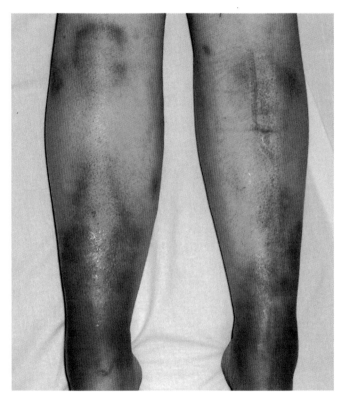

The CXR shows bilateral hilar lymphadenopathy and no consolidation.

U&E	normal
LFT	normal
Hb	12.5 g/dL
WCC	2.9×10^9/L
Lymphocytes	0.8×10^9/L
Platelets	368×10^9/L
Calcium	2.9 mmol/L
Albumin	37 g/L

1   What two investigations will be of most diagnostic value?

- [ ] A   Serum ACE
- [ ] B   Autoantibody screen
- [ ] C   ESR
- [ ] D   24-h urinary calcium
- [ ] E   Sputum microscopy and culture
- [ ] F   Bronchoalveolar lavage
- [ ] G   Mantoux test
- [ ] H   Biopsy of the rash
- [ ] I   HIV-antibody test
- [ ] J   High resolution CT of the chest

2   The most likely diagnosis is:

- [ ] A   Pulmonary tuberculosis
- [ ] B   Pulmonary histiocytosis X
- [ ] C   Histoplasmosis
- [ ] D   Sarcoidosis
- [ ] E   Lymphoma

Case 2

A 76-year-old lady is referred to hospital by her GP with a 48-hour history of profuse bloody diarrhoea associated with upper abdominal pain and fever. Other residents in her care home have developed a similar illness at the same time and the staff wonder if it is related to a meat pie – from a local butcher – that they had eaten 24–36 hours earlier. She has diet-controlled type 2 diabetes mellitus and hypertension. She had been reviewed in the diabetes clinic 2 weeks earlier. Her routine bloods were normal, HbA1$_c$ 6.5%. She takes lansoprazole 15 mg once daily and frusemide 40 mg once daily.

On examination she is confused (AMTS 5/10) with dry mucous membranes. Temperature is 36.2°C, pulse 100 bpm, blood pressure 100/50 mmHg, the JVP is not visible. She is tender to palpation in the epigastrium.

1   On the basis of the history, which three of the following would be most likely to be responsible?

☐   A   *Staphylococcus aureus*
☐   B   *Escherichia coli*
☐   C   *Bacillus cereus*
☐   D   *Vibrio parahaemolyticus*
☐   E   *Cryptosporidium parvum*
☐   F   *Campylobacter jejuni*
☐   G   *Salmonella*
☐   H   Rotavirus
☐   I   Norovirus
☐   J   *Clostridium difficile*

Urinalysis
Ketones   ++
Protein   +++
Red cells   ++++
White cells   +

Investigations:

Hb	9.7 g/dL
MCV	81 fL
WCC	7.6×10^9/L
Neutrophils	5.4×10^9/L
Platelets	41×10^9/L
Sodium	130 mmol/L
Potassium	5.8 mmol/L
Urea	26.2 mmol/L
Creatinine	224 µmol/L
Bicarbonate	19 mmol/L
Albumin	27 g/L
Glucose	18.5 mmol/L

2   Which one of the following is true?

- A She has diabetic ketoacidosis
- B An urgent blood film should be performed
- C Given the absence of a neutrophilia and fever the diarrhoea is probably not infectious in aetiology
- D The case should be notified to the public health department when a microbiological diagnosis is made
- E Her normal medications should be continued

3   Keeping the subsequent investigations in mind, the most likely cause is?

- A *Staphylococcus aureus*
- B *Escherichia coli*
- C *Bacillus cereus*
- D *Vibrio parahaemolyticus*
- E *Cryptosporidium parvum*
- F *Campylobacter jejuni*
- G *Salmonella* spp.
- H Rotavirus
- I Norovirus
- J *Clostridium difficile*

Case 3

A 28-year-old presents with a 2-day history of increasing headache and fever. On the evening of her admission she had not recognised her flat mate who had therefore called an ambulance. There is no relevant past medical history and she takes no regular medications. Her friend recalls that she had also complained of dysuria following her last sexual contact 6 weeks earlier.

On examination she is lethargic and drowsy. She has no rash. Temperature 37.9°C, pulse 100 bpm, blood pressure 105/60 mmHg. There is terminal neck stiffness and mild photophobia. The disc margins are clearly seen.

1   Which one of the following is true?

☐   A   The magnitude of the fever makes an acute HIV seroconversion illness unlikely

☐   B   The absence of rash makes meningococcal meningitis unlikely

☐   C   Drowsiness indicates involvement of the reticular activating formation in the brainstem

☐   D   A CT brain scan is not required before lumbar puncture

☐   E   Antibiotic treatment should be given before the lumbar puncture

A lumbar puncture is performed:

Opening pressure	18 cmH$_2$O
Protein	0.6 g/L
Glucose	3.7 mmol/L (plasma glucose 5.3 mmol/L)
WCC	95/mL (80% lymphocytes, 20% neutrophils)
RCC	<5/mL
Gram stain	negative

2   Which one of the following is the most appropriate empirical treatment?

☐   A   iv aciclovir and iv cefotaxime

☐   B   iv aciclovir

☐   C   iv ampicillin

☐   D   iv ciprofloxacin

☐   E   Symptomatic treatment only – analgesia, anti-emetics, fluids

An MRI brain scan is performed during her admission – see below.

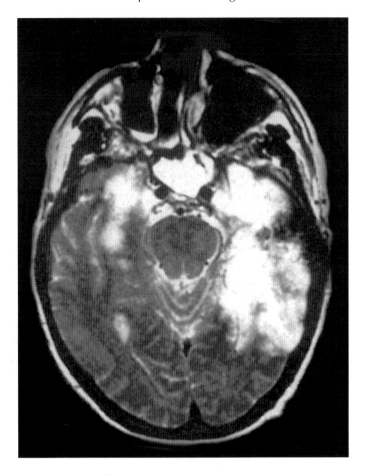

3   The most likely aetiological agent is:

- ☐ A   Varicella zoster virus (VZV)
- ☐ B   Herpes simplex virus 2 (HSV-2)
- ☐ C   *Listeria monocytogenes*
- ☐ D   Enterovirus
- ☐ E   *Neisseria gonorrhoeae*

Case 4

You are told about a 42-year-old oil engineer with a 3-day history of sore throat, fever, and rigors. His GP noticed an erythematous rash and bruising over the feet and has arranged an ambulance to your hospital. The symptoms had developed when he arrived home following a 6-week trip to rural Uganda. He did not take his malaria prophylaxis but was given the appropriate vaccinations by a travel clinic before his visit and he has a valid yellow fever vaccination certificate from 4 years ago.

1   Which one of the following statements is true?

☐   A   Clinical samples must be taken and analysed without delay
☐   B   He should be placed in a side room with negative pressure ventilation
☐   C   The Coombe's test will be positive
☐   D   HIV seroconversion is an unlikely differential diagnosis
☐   E   Yellow fever is an unlikely differential diagnosis

On arrival he looks unwell. Pulse is 100 bpm, blood pressure 120/65 mmHg, temperature 39.1°C. He has an erythematous pharynx. He is flushed with ecchymoses over the ankles but there is no specific rash. He has splenomegaly and is passing very dark urine (see below).

Investigations subsequently reveal:

Hb	7.9 g/dL
MCV	85 fL
WCC	4.5×10^9/L
Platelets	35×10^9/L
Sodium	135 mmol/L
Potassium	5.5 mmol/L
Urea	13.8 mmol/L
Creatinine	115 µmol/L
ALT	88 U/L
ALP	160 U/L
Bilirubin	40 µmol/L
PT	18 s
APTT	47 s
Fibrinogen	1.5 g/L

A malaria film (shown below) is reported as '5% parasitaemia. Species unknown'

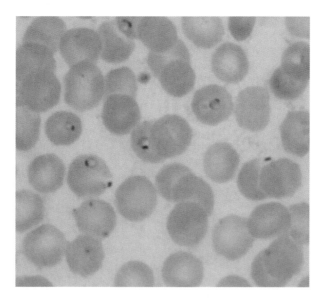

2   Which three of the following are true?

- [ ] A   iv quinine is contra-indicated if he has G6PD deficiency
- [ ] B   Treatment may be complicated by severe hypoglycaemia
- [ ] C   He will have lifelong immunity to future infection with this organism
- [ ] D   DIC is unlikely
- [ ] E   Initial treatment should be followed by oral primaquine
- [ ] F   The dark urine is the result of haematuria
- [ ] G   The infection can be transmitted via needlestick injury
- [ ] H   It is not a notifiable disease
- [ ] I   He has severe falciparum malaria

Case 5

A 42-year-old refugee presents with a 3-week history of increasing headache, fever, and confusion. He had arrived in the UK 4 weeks ago, having being smuggled into the country in a lorry driven across Europe from his home in Iraq. Before being assessed fully in A&E he has two generalised seizures of 1-min duration. He is given 2 mg lorazepam iv and is then unable to maintain his airway, so is intubated and transferred to the ITU.

On examination he is sedated, unconscious and is ventilated (closed circuit). Bilateral papilloedema is noted.

A CT brain is performed showing 'normal intracranial appearances'

CXR is 'Normal with an ET tube in situ'.

A lumbar puncture is then performed.

The CSF results are as follows:

Opening pressure	210 mmH$_2$O
Protein	2.8 g/L
Glucose	1.1 mmol/L
WCC	180/mL (70% lymphocytes, 30% neutrophils)
RCC	< 5/mL
Gram stain	negative
Ziehl-Neelsen stain	negative

1   Which is the most likely diagnosis?

- [ ] A   Cryptococcal meningitis
- [ ] B   Brucellosis
- [ ] C   Listeria meningitis
- [ ] D   Tuberculous meningitis
- [ ] E   CNS lymphoma

2   Which three of the following statements are true?

☐   A   An HIV antibody test can be performed without his consent
☐   B   The CT scan before lumbar puncture was unnecessary in this case
☐   C   As a refugee from outside of the EU he is not eligible for free medical treatment in this case
☐   D   He should be commenced on anti-epileptic medication
☐   E   He should be given iv mannitol
☐   F   An MRI scan may aid diagnosis
☐   G   Positive microbiological results must be obtained before commencing antimicrobials
☐   H   He must be nursed in a side room

Case 6

A 61-year-old married man is seen in the outpatient clinic with a several month history of epigastric pain, intermittent non-bloody diarrhoea, and weight loss. He was born in Jamaica and moved to the UK in the 1960s. He has not returned to Jamaica for many years. He admits to consuming 56 units alcohol per week. His GP arranged an OGD 4 months ago that was reported as showing 'mild gastritis'. He now takes lansoprazole but his symptoms persist. He also takes an antihistamine occasionally for an itchy rash on his trunk.

On examination he looks thin and unwell. There is nothing else of note.

Investigations reveal:

Hb	11.9 g/dL
MCV	90 fL
WCC	10.0×10^9/L
Neutrophils	7.0×10^9/L
Eosinophils	1.3×10^9/L
Platelets	160×10^9/L
Red cell folate	140 µmol/L

U&E	Normal
Calcium	2.05 mmol/L
Albumin	25 g/L
ALT	30 U/L
ALP	105 U/L
Bilirubin	2.1 µmol/L
Glucose	10.6 mmol/L
Amylase	95 U/L

A rigid sigmoidoscopy is performed in clinic. Histology shows inflammation of the submucosa. He is admitted for further investigations.

1   Which three of the following will be of most diagnostic value?

- ☐ A   Repeat gastroscopy with CLO test
- ☐ B   Jejunal biopsy
- ☐ C   String test
- ☐ D   Magnetic resonance cholangiopancreatography (MRCP)
- ☐ E   *Helicobacter pylori* serology
- ☐ F   Human T-cell leukaemia virus-1 (HTLV-1) serology
- ☐ G   Stool microscopy and culture
- ☐ F   Blood cultures
- ☐ G   Barium meal and follow through

2   What is the treatment of choice for this condition?

- ☐ A   iv ceftriaxone for 2 weeks
- ☐ B   Tinidazole 2 g orally
- ☐ C   Oral prednisolone and mesalazine
- ☐ D   *H. pylori* eradication therapy
- ☐ E   Ivermectin 200 µg/kg/day for 2 days

Case 7

A 26-year-old doctor presents with a 4-day history of fever and a blanching erythematous rash. A week earlier he returned from working in Kenya and Malawi for 6 months. He took appropriate malaria prophylaxis and used a mosquito net. He was given the appropriate vaccinations before his trip and drank bottled water. In the weeks before his return he had felt well and spent time sailing on Lake Malawi.

On examination he looks unwell. He is alert with no neck stiffness. Apart from a raised temperature of 38.1°C and a non-specific erythematous rash, examination is unremarkable.

Hb	14.7 g/dL
WCC	13.0×10^9/L
Eosinophils	1.6×10^9/L
Platelets	159×10^9/L
U&E	normal
LFT	normal
Schistosoma serology	negative
Malaria film	negative

1   Which of the following antimalarial prophylaxis regimens is inappropriate for Malawi?

- A   Doxycycline
- B   Chloroquine and proguanil
- C   Mefloquine
- D   Malarone (atovaquone-proguanil)
- E   Maloprim (pyrimethamine-dapsone)

2   Which one of the following will you exclude on the current information?

- A   Malaria
- B   Enteric fever
- C   Yellow fever
- D   Katayama fever (acute schistosomiasis)
- E   Dengue fever

His symptoms resolve and he returns to work. He presents several years later with per rectum bleeding and intermittent diarrhoea. Abdominal examination reveals nil of note. A stool examination reveals very occasional eggs, which are pictured below.

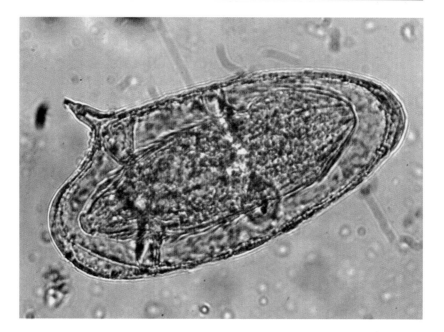

3   What organism is responsible for his symptoms?

☐ A   *Strongyloides stercoralis*
☐ B   *Trichinella spiralis*
☐ C   *Ancylostoma duodenale*
☐ D   *Ascaris lumbricoides*
☐ E   *Schistosoma mansoni*

Case 8

A 22-year-old student presents with a 2-week history of intermittent fever and upper abdominal pain. He had returned from backpacking across Asia and South-east Asia a month earlier. He took malaria prophylaxis and had the necessary vaccinations before travel. He is previously fit and well.

On examination he looks mildly unwell; pulse is 90 bpm, blood pressure 120/70 mmHg, temperature 37.4°C. In the abdomen there is tender 2-cm hepatomegaly.

Investigations:

Hb	11.7 g/dL
MCV	85 fL
WCC	14 × 10⁹/L
Neutrophils	11.1 × 10⁹/L
Eosinophils	0.3 × 10⁹/L
Platelets	170 × 10⁹/L
U&E	normal
Albumin	30 g/L
ALT	40 U/L
ALP	130 U/L
Bilirubin	18 µmol/L

Anti-HBs antibody >100 I/U

His ultrasound scan is shown below. The right lobe of the liver is shown. The remainder of the liver, kidneys, pancreas, and spleen were normal.

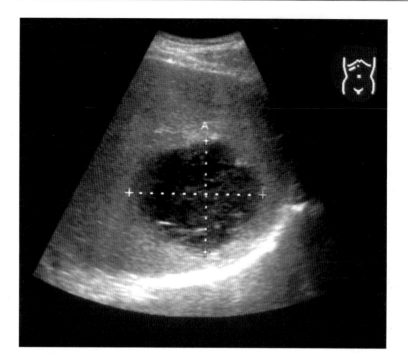

1   What is the likely diagnosis?

☐ A   Pyogenic liver abscess (PLA)
☐ B   Brucellosis
☐ C   Amoebic liver abscess (ALA)
☐ D   Hepatocellular carcinoma
☐ E   Hydatid disease

2   Which two of the following are the most useful diagnostic investigations?

☐ A   Microscopic examination of stool for ova, cysts, and parasites
☐ B   Stool culture
☐ C   Urine culture
☐ D   Blood culture
☐ E   Amoebic serology
☐ F   Hydatid serology
☐ G   Aspiration of abscess
☐ H   Serum alpha-fetoprotein (αFP)

Case 9

An 18-year-old student presents with 3 days of fever, headache, and anorexia. On the day of admission she developed neck pain and lower abdominal discomfort and was sent from the student health GP practice to the local hospital. She has no relevant previous medical history. She takes a combined oral contraceptive.

On examination she is febrile and looks unwell. The pulse is 112 bpm, and the blood pressure 105/75 mmHg. She has tender cervical lymphadenopathy and right facial swelling. The throat is clear and no rash is seen. The lower abdomen is tender but no discrete masses can be felt. She has mild terminal neck stiffness but no photophobia.

Investigations:

Hb	13.7 g/dL
MCV	80 fL
WCC	14.1×10^9/L
Platelets	245×10^9/L
LFT	normal

1   What is the likely diagnosis?

- A   Meningococcal meningitis
- B   Acute salpingitis
- C   Gonococcal infection
- D   Mumps
- E   Acute EBV infection

Case 10

A 40-year-old lady returns from Pakistan after visiting relatives. A week later she develops fever of slow onset, headache, myalgia, and a non-productive cough. Although she had a couple of episodes of diarrhoea while away she is now constipated. She took chloroquine for malaria prophylaxis.

On examination she looks unwell and depressed. The temperature is 37.9°C, pulse 60 bpm, the chest is clear. A tender 3-cm liver is palpated. No splenomegaly or rashes are found.

Investigations:

Hb	14.2 g/dL
WCC	3.2×10^9/L
Platelets	210×10^9/L
Albumin	28 g/L
ALT	75 U/L
ALP	115 U/L
Bilirubin	28 µmol/L

1   The next three most important investigations to be performed are:

- A   Malaria film
- B   Blood cultures
- C   Dengue serology
- D   Induced sputum
- E   Chest X-ray
- F   Hepatitis serology
- G   Atypical respiratory serology
- H   Abdominal ultrasound
- I   Widal test

Initial investigations are unhelpful. She is commenced on oral amoxicillin but her fever persists over the next 5 days. A urine culture identifies a Gram negative organism.

2   The antibiotics should be changed to:

- A   Oral ciprofloxacin
- B   iv chloramphenicol
- C   Oral doxycycline
- D   Oral trimethoprim
- E   iv augmentin
- F   No change in antibiotics

3 **Which one of the following statements is true?**

☐ A The infection does not resolve spontaneously
☐ B Fulminant liver failure often occurs in untreated disease
☐ C Lifelong immunity occurs after infection
☐ D Serology is the most reliable test
☐ E Bone marrow aspiration and culture is a useful diagnostic test

Case 11

A 24-year-old soldier returns from Belize where he was stationed for several weeks. He took part in army exercises in the local jungle. He developed a skin lesion on his left foot after returning to the UK.

The picture shows the lesion 3 weeks after onset.

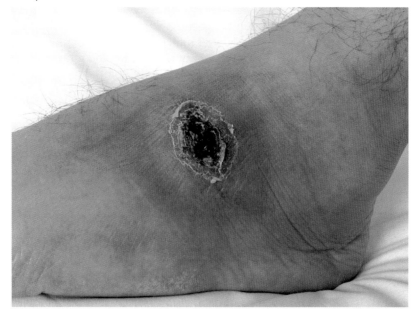

His blood tests are all normal.

1   What is the organism responsible?

- A   *Ancylostoma brasiliensis*
- B   *Mycobacterium ulcerans*
- C   *Trypanosoma cruzi*
- D   *Leishmania braziliensis*
- E   *Paracoccidioidomycosis brasiliensis*

Case 12

A 28-year-old man presents with a 2-day history of fever, headache, rash, and severe arthralgia. He returned from a 2-day business trip to India 4 days before the onset of symptoms. He recalls several mosquito bites but had not taken malaria prophylaxis – he moved to the UK from India 4 months ago and did not feel prophylaxis was necessary.

On examination he is conscious and alert. Temperature is 37.8°C, pulse 100 bpm, blood pressure 105/65 mmHg. He has a maculopapular rash on his trunk and limbs that blanches to pressure and mild right upper quadrant tenderness. There is nothing else of note.

Initial blood test reveals:

Hb	14.7 g/dL
WCC	2.4 × 10⁹/L
Lymphocytes	1.5 × 10⁹/L
Platelets	42 × 10⁹/L
U&E	normal
Albumin	37 g/L
ALT	90 U/L
ALP	105 U/L
Bilirubin	28 μmol/L
Malaria antibody	positive
CXR	normal

1   The most likely diagnosis is:

☐   A   Yellow fever
☐   B   Falciparum malaria
☐   C   Acute hepatitis A
☐   D   Acute HIV infection
☐   E   Dengue fever

Case 13

A 25-year-old masseuse presents with a productive cough, myalgia, and fever. CXR reveals left basal consolidation; iv cefuroxime and oral erythromycin are commenced. Her symptoms improve and her fever resolves, however, 5 days after admission she develops left-sided chest pain and increasing shortness of breath.

On examination her temperature is 37.7°C and she has reduced air entry at the left base. Her CXR is shown below.

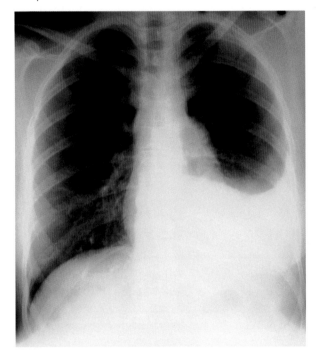

A diagnostic pleural aspiration is performed:

Cell count	12 × 10⁹/L (neutrophils)
pH	7.28
LDH	750 U/L
Protein	30 g/L
Glucose	4.1 mmol/L
Gram stain	negative

Blood tests reveal:

Serum protein	56 g/L
Serum LDH	700 U/L

1   Which of the following is correct?

☐ A   She has a simple parapneumonic effusion
☐ B   She has an empyema
☐ C   The effusion is a transudate
☐ D   A pulmonary embolus is unlikely
☐ E   An intercostal chest drain should be inserted

While taking a further history, the patient mentions to you that she had visited a petting zoo with her niece 3 weeks before her symptoms began.

2   What is the most likely diagnosis?

☐ A   Leptospirosis
☐ B   Brucellosis
☐ C   Nocardia pneumonia
☐ D   Q fever
☐ E   Psittacosis

Case 14

An injecting heroin user presents with a painful, swollen left arm. He had recently been injecting into veins in his upper arm and had presented to A&E 36 hours ago with severe arm pain. The SHO had noted a 'mildly red arm' and the patient was discharged with oral flucloxacillin.

On examination he looks unwell. Temperature is 38.8°C, pulse 140 pm, blood pressure 95/65 mmHg. His arm is pictured below.

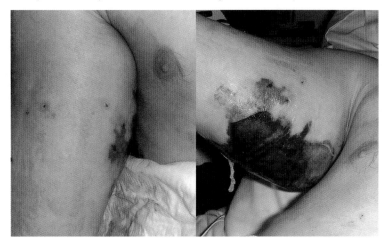

1   Which two of the following are true?

- [ ] A   He should be resuscitated then taken to theatre
- [ ] B   Daily operations will be required
- [ ] C   Antibiotics should be changed to include iv flucloxacillin and iv penicillin
- [ ] D   Hyperbaric oxygen therapy may be of benefit
- [ ] E   The most likely causative organism is a group B streptococcus
- [ ] F   Central venous access should be avoided given his concurrent heroin use
- [ ] G   Drotrecogin-alpha is contra-indicated

Case 15

A 47-year-old lady returns from a cruise down the River Amazon with a large boil on her arm. Her GP prescribes flucloxacillin with no benefit. She presents to A&E where an SHO attempts to incise and drain the lesion. However, the organism shown below is extracted instead.

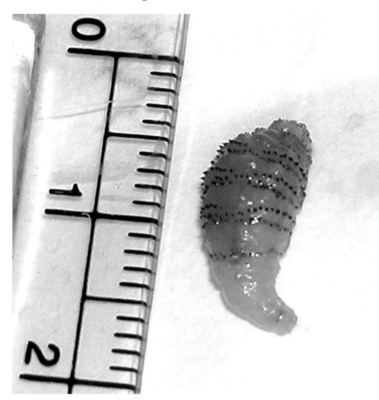

1   What is this?

- [ ] A   *Ancylostoma braziliense*
- [ ] B   *Chrysomyia* larva (screw worm)
- [ ] C   Tumbu fly larva
- [ ] D   Bot fly larva
- [ ] E   *Tunga penetrans* (chigger)
- [ ] F   Guinea worm (Dracunculiasis)

Case 16

A 35-year-old woman is found collapsed at home by her husband. She had been unwell with a 12-h history of fever and myalgia. Before the collapse she had developed non-bloody diarrhoea. There is no previous medical history of note. Her GP had recently changed her oral contraceptive to an intrauterine contraceptive device.

On examination she is drowsy. The temperature is 39.1 °C, pulse 120 bpm, blood pressure 87/40 mmHg; the chest is clear, abdominal and pelvic examination reveals nothing of note. She has no meningism. A widespread, confluent erythematous rash is seen affecting all areas.

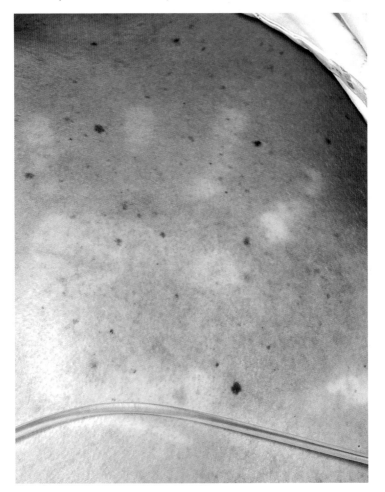

Investigations:

Hb	13.1 g/dL
WCC	14.7×10^9/L
Neutrophils	12.4×10^9/L
Platelets	95×10^9/L
Sodium	134 mmol/L
Potassium	5.9 mmol/L
Urea	18.7 mmol/L
Creatinine	228 µmol/L
Bicarbonate	16 mmol/L
ALT	95 U/L
ALP	85 U/L
Bilirubin	30 µmol/L
CK	455 U/L

1   The most likely causative organism is:

- [ ] A   *Staphylococcus aureus*
- [ ] B   *Pseudomonas aeruginosa*
- [ ] C   *Streptococcus pneumoniae*
- [ ] D   *Neisseria meningitidis*
- [ ] E   *Neisseria gonorrhoeae*

Despite resuscitation with iv fluids her systolic blood pressure remains below 90 mmHg. Her oxygen saturations fall and auscultation of the chest reveals bibasal crepitations.

2   Immediate management involves which one of the following:

- [ ] A   Parenteral glucocorticoids
- [ ] B   Pooled platelet transfusion to keep the count about 100×10^9/l
- [ ] C   Consideration of drotrecogin-alpha therapy
- [ ] D   Broad spectrum antibiotics with anti-pseudomanal cover
- [ ] E   Lumbar puncture and examination of CSF

Case 17

A 55-year-old retired engineer presents with a several-month history of lethargy, weight loss, and abdominal discomfort. He spends most of the year outside the UK, residing in Malta, and admits to drinking several gin and tonics daily. Earlier in the year a gastroenterologist had reviewed him. Blood tests at that time revealed a normocytic anaemia and deranged LFT. Ultrasound of the abdomen revealed hepatosplenomegaly. A diagnosis of alcoholic liver disease was made.

On examination he looks thin and pale. Temperature is 37.6°C; he has 3-cm hepatomegaly and 8-cm splenomegaly.

Blood tests reveal:

Hb	9.4 g/dL
MCV	96 fL
WCC	2.5×10^9/L
Neutrophils	0.9×10^9/L
Platelets	80×10^9/L
PT	16 s
Albumin	24 g/L
ALT	80 U/L
ALP	140 U/L
Bilirubin	17 μmol/L

A bone marrow biopsy is shown overleaf.

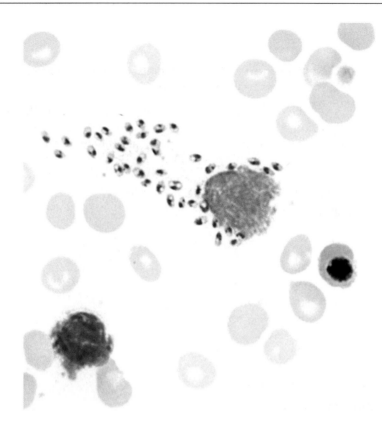

1   Which one of the following is the correct diagnosis

☐ A   Chronic disseminated histoplasmosis
☐ B   Chronic lymphocytic leukaemia
☐ C   Alcoholic liver disease
☐ D   Visceral leishmaniasis
☐ E   Non-Hodgkin's lymphoma

Case 18

A 15-year-old boy presents with a sore throat and fever. He has recently arrived in the UK with his family from Ukraine.

On examination he looks unwell. Temperature is 38.0°C, pulse 68 bpm and blood pressure 95/60 mmHg. Examination of the throat reveals an exudative pharyngitis, the thick green exudate extending onto the palate. He has cervical lymphadenopathy. A soft systolic murmur is heard at the left sternal edge. He has a hoarse voice and a thick neck but his parents cannot say if these are new signs.

Lead II from his ECG is illustrated below.

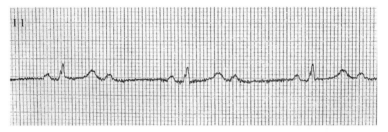

1 The most likely diagnosis is:

☐ A   Rheumatic fever
☐ B   Miller–Fisher syndrome
☐ C   Diphtheria
☐ D   Congo-Crimean haemorrhagic fever (CCHF)
☐ E   *Fusobacterium necrophorum* infection (Lemierre's syndrome)

2 Which one of the following will be of most benefit to the patient?

☐ A   iv immunoglobulin
☐ B   iv benzylpenicillin
☐ C   Transfer to CCU
☐ D   iv diphtheria anti-toxin
☐ E   iv ribavarin

Case 19

A 20-year-old man presents with 2 weeks of fatigue and a tender left axilla. He is a second-year veterinary student and has had several girlfriends since he began university.

On examination he looks well and is afebrile. He has large, tender left axillary lymphadenopathy. The overlying skin is red and one of the nodes is suppurative. There are no lesions on the left arm. He has small inguinal lymph nodes.

1   Which one of the following is the most likely cause?

- ☐   A   *Francisella tularensis*
- ☐   B   *Chlamydia trachomatis*
- ☐   C   *Bartonella henselae*
- ☐   D   *Bacillus anthracis*
- ☐   E   *Capnocytophaga canimorsus*

Case 20

*A 29-year-old single man presents with headache and jaundice. This
followed a 5-day history of fever, headache, and severe myalgia. He
had assumed these symptoms were the result of a 'cold' picked up
during a canoeing trip to North Wales (his brother's 'stag do') 1 week
earlier, as they were beginning to resolve.*

On examination he looks unwell. He has jaundiced sclera with marked
conjunctival injection. Temperature is 38.1°C, pulse 100 bpm and
blood pressure 96/60 mmHg. The chest is clear. A tender liver is just
palpable beneath the right costal margin. He has scattered crepitations
on auscultation of the chest and neck stiffness.

Investigations:

Hb	12.9 g/dL
WCC	14.1 × 10⁹/L
Neutrophils	12.2 × 10⁹/L
Platelets	80 × 10⁹/L
Sodium	135 mmol/L
Potassium	5.1 mmol/L
Urea	16.7 mmol/L
Creatinine	185 mmol/L
Albumin	25 g/L
ALT	145 U/L
ALP	110 U/L
Bilirubin	59 µmol/L

1   Which one of the following is the most likely diagnosis?

- [ ] A Acute hepatitis A
- [ ] B Acute hepatitis B
- [ ] C Leptospirosis
- [ ] D Meningococcal meningitis
- [ ] E Legionella pneumonia

Case 21

A 26-year-old woman presents to hospital following a generalised seizure. She has a long history of repeated hospital admissions since childhood. She is on no regular medication.

On examination she is conscious and alert. Temperature is 37.9°C. You notice the appearance of her hands (see below). Auscultation of the heart reveals an ejection systolic murmur associated with a thrill. She has reduced power in her right upper limb with reduced reflexes.

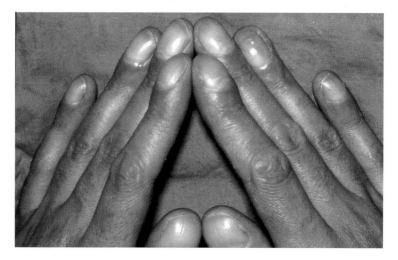

MRI and CT scans of the brain are subsequently performed.

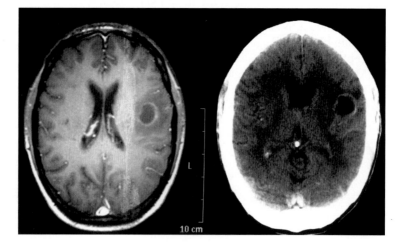

10 cm

Blood results:

Hb	19.6 g/dL
MCV	88 fL
WCC	16.7×10^9/L
Neutrophils	14.8×10^9/L
Lymphocytes	1.5×10^9/L
Platelets	160×10^9/L

1   Which three investigations would be of most diagnostic value?

☐ A   Blood cultures
☐ B   Transthoracic echocardiogram (TTE)
☐ C   Lumbar puncture
☐ D   Stereotactic brain biopsy
☐ E   HIV antibody test
☐ F   Toxoplasma serology
☐ G   CXR
☐ H   CD4 lymphocyte count

2   Which one of the following is the most likley diagnosis?

☐ A   Astrocytoma
☐ B   Toxoplasma meningoencephalitis
☐ C   Tuberculoma
☐ D   Cerebral abscess
☐ E   Cerebral lymphoma

Case 22

You are asked to see a 35-year-old injecting drug user in A&E. He had presented with jaw pain and difficulty in swallowing earlier that day. He was sent away with oral penicillin. Later that day he was brought in by ambulance following a respiratory arrest in the street. This had not responded to iv naloxone and he had been intubated. Marked muscular rigidity made ventilation difficult, and large doses of midazolam were given.

He is now mechanically ventilated. There is little to find on examination except for the skin lesions on the patient's limbs as shown below (inset shows close up).

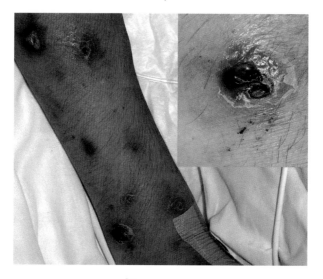

1   Which one of the following is the most likley diagnosis?

- [ ] A   Botulism
- [ ] B   Diphtheria
- [ ] C   Crack cocaine encephalopathy
- [ ] D   Guillain–Barré syndrome
- [ ] E   Tetanus

2   Further management includes which two of the following:

☐   A   iv immunoglobulin
☐   B   Nursing in a quiet environment
☐   C   Human anti-tetanus immunoglobulin
☐   D   iv clofazamine
☐   E   Botulinum anti-toxin
☐   F   Plasma exchange
☐   G   Treatment of autonomic dysfunction with plasma expanders and/or cardiac glycosides
☐   H   Lumbar puncture and examination of CSF

Case 23

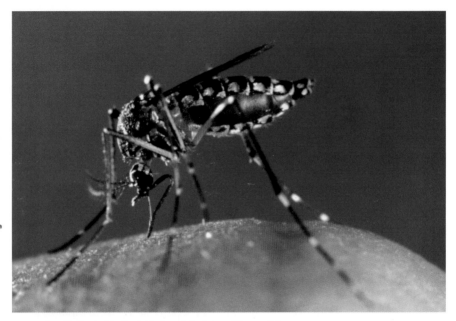

Credit: Jack K. Clark/AgStock/Science Photo, Library.

1   The above insect is associated with transmission of which seven of the following:

- ☐ A   Yellow fever virus
- ☐ B   *Wuchereria bancrofti*
- ☐ C   *Leishmania* spp.
- ☐ D   Dengue virus
- ☐ E   *Borrelia burgdorferi*
- ☐ F   *Trypanosoma cruzi*
- ☐ G   *Trypanosoma brucei*
- ☐ H   *Onchocerca volvulus*
- ☐ I   *Borrelia recurrentis*
- ☐ J   Japanese encephalitis virus
- ☐ K   *Brugia malayi*
- ☐ L   Lassa fever virus
- ☐ M   Ebola virus
- ☐ N   *Rickettsia rickettsii*
- ☐ O   *Loa loa*
- ☐ P   West Nile virus
- ☐ Q   *Plasmodium malariae*
- ☐ R   Hantaviruses

Case 24

A 24-year-old lady presents with a 3-day history of increasing breathlessness. A week earlier while on a hill-walking holiday she had a flu-like illness that resolved.

On examination she is short of breath at rest, the pulse is 120 bpm, blood pressure 100/70 mmHg and the JVP 6 cm. Auscultation reveals a soft systolic murmur and a third heart sound together with bibasal crepitations.

FBC, U&E, LFT   all normal
Troponin I   4.5 ng/ml

Below is her ECG

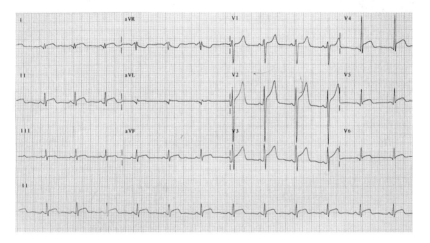

1   What is the most likely diagnosis?

☐ A   Rheumatic fever
☐ B   Acute viral myocarditis
☐ C   Hypertrophic obstructive cardiomyopathy
☐ D   Dilated cardiomyopathy
☐ E   Lyme disease

Case 25

A 28-year old man develops fever, general malaise, and a dry cough. He has acute myeloid leukaemia and received an allogeneic bone marrow transplant 7 days ago. He has been taking fluconazole 100 mg od, valaciclovir 500 mg od, and ciprofloxacin 500 mg od for 2 weeks.

On examination he looks moderately unwell. The temperature is 38.2°C, pulse 120 bpm, blood pressure 105/80 mmHg. His lips and oropharynx are inflamed but no ulceration is seen; his chest is clear; he has palpable hepatosplenomegaly. No rash is seen. His Hickman line (tunnelled intravascular catheter) site looks clean.

Investigations:

U&E and LFT	normal.
Hb	9.4 g/dL
MCV	95 fL
WCC	1.1×10^9/L
Neutrophils	0.2×10^9/L
Lymphocytes	0.6×10^9/L
Platelets	22×10^9/L
CXR	Hickman line in situ

1   Which empirical antibiotic regimen should be commenced?

- [ ] A   iv cefotaxime and erythromycin
- [ ] B   iv ciprofloxacin
- [ ] C   iv vancomycin
- [ ] D   iv tazocin – (piperacillin and tazobactam)
- [ ] E   Linezolid po

2   Which of the following is true?

- [ ] A   Empirical antibiotics have yet to be shown to reduce mortality in this setting
- [ ] B   A source of infection is only found in one third of cases afer a thorough search
- [ ] C   Antibiotics can be discontinued with defervescence
- [ ] D   Granulocyte transfusion should be considered at this stage
- [ ] E   Graft-versus-host disease (GVHD) is unlikely

His fever persists over the next 4 days and his neutrophil count remains 0.2×10^9/L. Examination reveals extensive inflammation of the oral mucosa. The skin around the Hickman line site is red. There are no positive culture results.

3   Which one of the following is true?

☐   A   An iv glycopeptide should be added to the regimen
☐   B   Cytomegalovirus (CMV) reactivation is likely
☐   C   A persisting fever indicates failure of antibiotic treatment
☐   D   Antifungal therapy should only be used following positive culture
          results
☐   E   The Hickman line should be replaced

Case 26

An 18-year-old university student presents with a 4-day history of fever, sore throat, abdominal discomfort, and cervical lymphadenopathy. He had arrived at university 6 weeks earlier and had quickly found a new girlfriend.

On examination he has a temperature of 38.9°C, widespread lymphadenopathy, a faint macular rash, and hepatosplenomegaly.

Blood tests reveal:

Hb	14.7 g/dL
WCC	19.8 × 10⁹/L
Lymphocytes	13.8 × 10⁹/L
Platelets	320 × 10⁹/L
Albumin	38 g/L
ALT	280 U/L
ALP	130 U/L
Bilirubin	28 μmol/L
Hepatitis B cAb	positive
Monospot test	negative
EBV VCA IgM	positive

1   Which one of the following is the most likely diagnosis?

☐ A   Acute hepatitis B
☐ B   Acute hepatitis C
☐ C   Acute HIV infection
☐ D   Epstein–Barr virus infection
☐ E   Cytomegalovirus infection

2   Which of the following is true?

☐ A   His girlfriend requires blood tests to exclude infection
☐ B   He is now excluded from donating blood
☐ C   He should avoid contact sports for at least 1 month
☐ D   Barrier contraception should be advised
☐ E   A notification form should be sent to the HPA

Case 27

A 42-year-old presents with a 4-day history of fever and a dry cough. He and his wife returned from a caving expedition to France and Spain 3 weeks earlier.

On examination he looks only mildly unwell. The temperature is 37.8°C. Oxygen saturations are 96% on air. Auscultation of the chest reveals scattered crepitations.

His CXR is shown below:

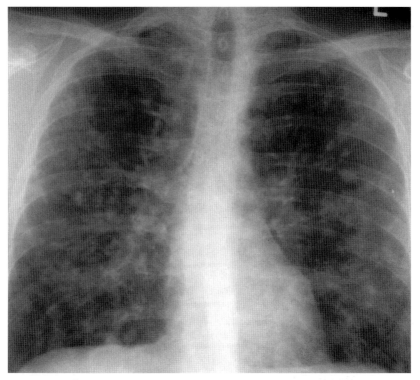

For image reference, see page viii

1   Which one of the following is the most likely diagnosis?

- [ ] A   Sarcoidosis
- [ ] B   Legionella pneumonia
- [ ] C   *Pneumocystis carinii* (*P. jiroveci*) pneumonia
- [ ] D   Miliary tuberculosis
- [ ] E   Acute pulmonary histoplasmosis

Case 28

A 21-year-old returns to the UK from a backpacking holiday to South-east Asia including Vietnam and Thailand. She presents with progressive weight loss, intermittent fevers, and a productive cough. There is no significant past medical history.

On examination she is thin, temperature is 37.9°C. Auscultation of the chest reveals left mid-zone crepitations (see CXR below). A gram negative rod is cultured from her sputum.

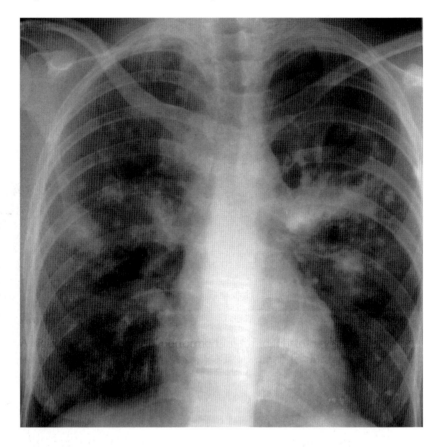

1   Which one of the following is the likely cause of her illness?

- [ ] A   *Mycobacterium tuberculosis*
- [ ] B   *Burkholderia pseudomallei*
- [ ] C   *Penicillium marneffei*
- [ ] D   *Cryptococcus neoformans*
- [ ] E   *Pseudomonas aeruginosa*

Case 29

A 61-year-old man presents with a 2-month history of weight loss, cough, and haemoptysis. He recalls being treated for tuberculosis as a teenager when in India. He then moved to the UK. He is a lifelong smoker.

On examination he is thin. You wonder if he shows clubbing of the fingers. The temperature is 37.3°C. Auscultation reveals occasional right mid-zone crepitations.

Bloods tests:

Hb	10.7 g/dL
MCV	85 fl
WCC	10.6 × 10⁹/L
Lymphocytes	1.2 × 10⁹/L
Platelets	410 × 10⁹/L

Aspergillus precipitins	negative
Galactomannan test	negative

CXR shows cavitating lung lesion in right upper zone.

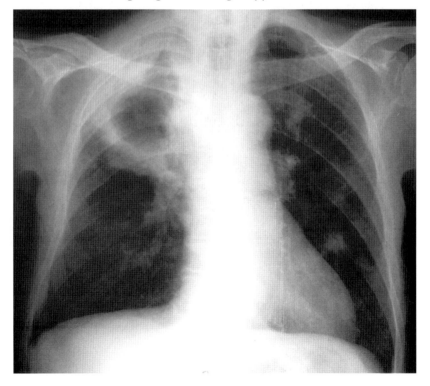

1   Which one of the following is the most likely diagnosis?

☐   A   Relapse of pulmonary tuberculosis
☐   B   Re-infection with *M. tuberculosis*
☐   C   Aspergilloma
☐   D   Invasive aspergillosis
☐   E   Squamous cell carcinoma of lung

Case 30

A 59-year-old woman is planning a 4-week holiday to Kenya with her husband in a few months time. She moved from Kenya to the UK 20 years ago but has not returned since then. She suffers with rheumatoid arthritis and depression. Her current medication includes methotrexate 1.5 mg weekly, prednisolone 4 mg daily, and citalopram 20 mg once daily.

1   **Which one of the following choices could be recommended for malaria prevention?**

- [ ] A   No chemoprophylaxis as she is immune to malaria
- [ ] B   Mefloquine 250 mg weekly
- [ ] C   Chloroquine 300 mg weekly with proguanil 200 mg daily
- [ ] D   Quinine 300 mg daily
- [ ] E   Doxycycline 100 mg daily

2   **Which three of the following vaccinations are recommended for this patient?**

- [ ] A   Oral polio
- [ ] B   Diphtheria and tetanus toxoid
- [ ] C   Yellow fever
- [ ] D   Injectable typhoid
- [ ] E   Hepatitis A
- [ ] F   Hepatitis B

Case 31

A patient returns from a camping holiday in South Africa with a lesion on her leg (shown below). She did not recall any bites but her travelling companions had removed several insects from their skin. She had a mild 'flu-like' illness while there but is now well.

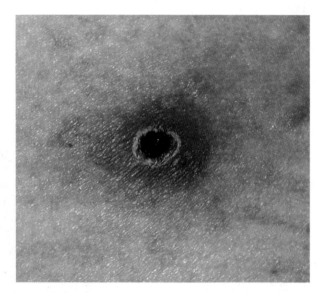

1 **Which one of the following is the most likely diagnosis?**

☐ A Anthrax (*Bacillus anthracis*)
☐ B Plague (*Yersinia pestis*)
☐ C African tick-bite fever (*Rickettsia africae*)
☐ D Lymes disease (*Borrelia burgdorferi*)
☐ E Tularaemia (*Francisella tularensis*)

Case 32

A 24-year-old man presents with a 24-hour history of fever and increasing shortness of breath. He had been involved in a road traffic accident 12 months earlier in Europe and underwent a splenectomy. He cannot recall any vaccinations given at the time and is on no regular medication.

On examination he is drowsy, the temperature is 39.5°C, pulse 120 bpm and blood pressure 90/55 mmHg. Arterial O_2 saturation is 95% on 6 litres O_2. Auscultation of the chest reveals bibasal crepitations. There is no neck stiffness or rash.

His CXR is shown below.

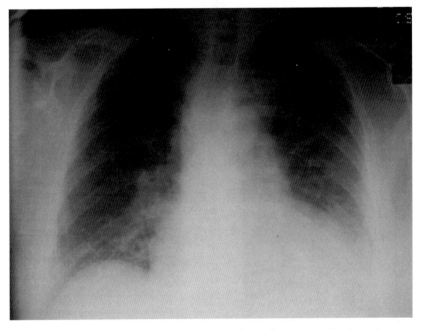

Image reproduced with permission from Dr Alexandra Nanzer, Registrar in Respiratory Medicine, Newham University Hospital.

1   Which three of the following are appropriate in his initial management?

☐ A   Induced sputum for urgent Ziehl–Neelsen stain and PCP PCR
☐ B   Plasma CMV (cytomegalovirus) IgG and PCR
☐ C   CT brain followed by lumbar puncture
☐ D   Intravenous broad-spectrum antibiotics
☐ E   Transfer to high dependency unit
☐ F   Aggressive fluid resuscitation
☐ G   iv co-trimoxazole
☐ H   iv gancyclovir

He recovers and is ready for discharge from hospital. You must counsel him and arrange appropriate management.

2   Which of following is true?

☐ A   He does not require long-term antibiotic prophylaxis
☐ B   Aminoglycosides should be avoided in this patient
☐ C   He should not receive either pneumococcal and *Haemophilus influenzae* type B immunisations.
☐ D   He should receive meningococcal group C vaccination
☐ E   He is protected against severe malaria

Case 33

A 35-year-old lady is referred to clinic by her GP with a persistent 'runny nose'. This followed a head injury 8 weeks ago associated with loss of consciousness.

On examination she has a clear discharge from both nostrils.

Further analysis reveals:

Protein	0.4 g/L
Glucose	4.1 mmol/L
RCC	<5/mL
WCC	2/mL

1   Further management includes which of the following?

- ☐ A   Lumbar puncture and blood patch
- ☐ B   Daily prophylactic antibiotics
- ☐ C   Neurosurgical repair with cadaveric dural graft
- ☐ D   Teriparatide followed by cyclical bisphosphonates
- ☐ E   *Haemophilus influenzae* B vaccination

Case 34

A 27-year-old woman presents to A&E with a 1-day history of headache, vomiting, and fever. She is on no medication. On transfer to hospital in an ambulance there was one witnessed tonic-clonic seizure that was quickly terminated with rectal diazepam.

On examination the temperature is 38.8°C, GCS is 14/15 and she is confused. There is no evidence of a rash or neck stiffness.

1   Which one of the following is the likely diagnosis?

☐   A   Varicella zoster encephalitis
☐   B   Sagittal sinus thrombosis
☐   C   Bacterial meningitis
☐   D   Brain abscess
☐   E   Herpes simplex encephalitis

2   What investigation of choice would confirm the diagnosis?

☐   A   MRI brain
☐   B   CSF culture
☐   C   Blood cultures
☐   D   CSF PCR
☐   E   EEG

Case 35

A 19-year-old student is admitted for investigation of intermittent fever, night sweats, and marked lower back pain. Two weeks ago she returned from her gap year trekking round the world.

On examination the temperature is 39.5°C and there is palpable hepatosplenomegaly, urinalysis is normal.

Investigations:

Hb	9.9 g/dL
WCC	3.2 × 10⁹/L
Neutrophils	1.5 × 10⁹/L
Platelets	100 × 10⁹/L
Sodium	142 mmol/L
Potassium	3.9 mmol/L
Urea	6.0 mmol/L
Creatinine	85 µmol/L
Bilirubin	18 µmol/L
AST	247 U/L
ALP	70 U/L
Albumin	29 U/L
CRP	80 mg/L

Urine β-HCG   negative

1   Which one of the following is the investigation of choice for imaging?

A   MRI spine
B   Spine X-ray
C   Bone scan
D   CT spine
E   Myelogram

2   What test would most accurately confirm the diagnosis?

A   Blood cultures
B   Bone marrow culture
C   Acute and convalescent serology
D   Liver biopsy
E   Mantoux test

Case 36

A 42-year-old lady originally from Kenya, presents with a 6-month history of central abdominal pain, nausea, diarrhoea, and intermittent fevers with a 1-day history of vomiting. She has lost 10 kg in weight. She takes no medication, and does not drink alcohol.

On examination she is thin, the temperature is 36.5°C, there is no jaundice and no hepatosplenomegaly. A mass is felt in the right iliac fossa, and shifting dullness is elicited.

Investigations:

Hb	9.3 g/dL
WCC	3.8 × 10⁹/L
Neutrophils	1.6 × 10⁹/L
Platelets	120 × 10⁹/L
Sodium	134 mmol/L
Potassium	4.8 mmol/L
Urea	3.6 mmol/L
Creatinine	81 µmol/L
Bilirubin	12 µmol/L
AST	65 U/L
ALP	165 U/L
Albumin	24 U/L
CRP	20 mg/L
CA-125	60 U/ml
CXR	normal
AXR	no colonic dilatation

1   Which one of the following is the most likely diagnosis?

- A   Crohn's disease
- B   Ovarian tumour
- C   Primary biliary cirrhosis
- D   Tuberculosis
- E   Ileocaecal adenocarcinoma

2   What test would you do to confirm your diagnosis?

- A   Colonoscopy plus biopsy
- B   Laporoscopy
- C   Ascitic paracentesis
- D   Faecal occult blood
- E   Ultrasound-guided biopsy

Case 37

A 47-year-old man is admitted for investigation of a rapid-onset acute confusional state associated with a 6-day history of intermittent fever and a 2-day history of diarrhoea and headache. His wife states that he came back from a business trip to the Ivory Coast 10 days ago. He rapidly deteriorates on arrival in A&E and is moved to the resuscitation room.

On examination: he is febrile, temperature 39.2°C, GCS 3/15, heart rate 140 bpm, blood pressure 90/50 mmHg, chest clear, abdomen no abnormality detected. No neck stiffness or rash.

Investigations reveal:

Hb	9.5 g/dL
WCC	15.8 × 10⁹/L
Neutrophils	14.0 × 10⁹/L
Platelets	88 × 10⁹/L
Sodium	134 mmol/L
Potassium	6.3 mmol/L
Urea	37.5 mmol/L
Creatinine	310 µmol/L
Bilirubin	70 µmol/L
AST	150 U/L
ALP	120 U/L
Albumin	34 U/L
CRP	78 mg/L

1   What management plan will you initiate?

- [ ] A   ITU referral, intubation, central-line insertion, iv ceftriaxone
- [ ] B   ITU referral, intubation, central-line insertion, iv ciprofloxacin, fluid resuscitation
- [ ] C   ITU referral, intubation, central-line insertion, iv quinine, haemofiltration
- [ ] D   ITU referral, intubation, central-line insertion, iv ciprofloxacin, haemofiltration
- [ ] E   ITU referral, intubation, central-line insertion, iv quinine, iv hydrocortisone, haemofiltration

Case 38

A 29-year-old man originally from Estonia presents with a 3-week history of productive cough and fevers. CXR demonstrates a left pleural effusion. Urgent sputum staining for AFB is negative.

You commence treatment for pulmonary tuberculosis with rifampacin, isoniazid, pyrazinamide, and ethambutol. You counsel him for an HIV test, which is negative.

You review the patient in clinic after 6 weeks of rifampicin, isoniazid, pyrazinamide, and ethambutol. The fevers have improved, but still persist, and he still has a productive cough.

Sputum culture at 35 days isolated *Mycobacterium tuberculosis*.

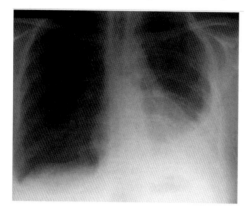

1   What do you do next?

- [ ] A   Repeat the CXR
- [ ] B   Send isolate to Reference Laboratory
- [ ] C   Start steroids
- [ ] D   Arrange for directly observed therapy (DOT)
- [ ] E   Check the urine

Case 39

A 45-year-old man presents with a 4-day history of fatigue, fever, vomiting, abdominal pain, and myalgia in his legs. He has had no foreign travel in the last 2 years and works as a plumber. He is married with a 2-year-old son; the family are well.

On examination his temperature is 39.2°C, he is jaundiced, the heart rate is 108 bpm, blood pressure is 130/90 mmHg, hearts sound are normal, and there are no murmurs; the chest is clear; in the abdomen there are no palpable organs, there is mild right upper quadrant tenderness. CNS examination reveals no focal neurology.

Urinalysis

Protein	+++
Blood	++
Leukocytes	negative
Glucose	negative

Investigations reveal:

Hb	11.7 g/dL
WCC	11.0×10^9/L
Neutrophils	9.7×10^9/L
Platelets	190×10^9/L
Sodium	141 mmol/L
Potassium	4.7 mmol/L
Urea	7.8 mmol/L
Creatinine	110 μmol/L
Bilirubin	80 μmol/L
AST	150 U/L
ALP	380 U/L
Albumin	32 U/L

1   Which one of the following is the likely diagnosis?

- [ ] A   Acute hepatitis B infection
- [ ] B   Acute hepatitis C infection
- [ ] C   Typhoid fever
- [ ] D   Malaria
- [ ] E   Leptospirosis

Case 40

A 48-year-old women presents with a fever and diarrhoea. She is 8 weeks post renal transplantation.

On examination, the temperature is 38.3°C, the heart rate is 100 bpm, blood pressure 115/60 mmHg, the chest is clear, the abdomen shows generalised discomfort, there is no focal graft tenderness. There are no focal CNS signs.

Urinalysis

protein   +

Investigations:

Hb	9.3 g/dL
WCC	2.0×10^9/L
Neutrophils	1.6×10^9/L
Platelets	240×10^9/L
Sodium	135 mmol/L
Potassium	4.0 mmol/L
Urea	8.8 mmol/L
Creatinine	120 µmol/L
Bilirubin	11 µmol/L
AST	130 U/L
ALP	50 U/L
Albumin	32 U/L
CRP	15 mg/L

1   What is the most likely cause of her fever?

- ☐ A   Acute CMV infection
- ☐ B   Acute graft-versus-host disease
- ☐ C   *Clostridium difficile* infection
- ☐ D   *Cryptosporidium parvum* infection
- ☐ E   Parvovirus B19 infection

Case 41

A 33-year-old women presents with a fever and acute confusion. She has recently been on a 10-day holiday to the Philippines where she was complaining of lethargy and bloody diarrhoea.

On examination: temperature 39.9°C, GCS 14/15, HR 110 bpm, blood pressure 135/70 mmHg, the chest is clear, the abdomen has generalised tenderness and discomfort, a pink rash is noted on the abdomen, no focal neurology in the CNS.

1   What treatment will you commence?

- ☐ A   Metronidazole
- ☐ B   Chloroquine
- ☐ C   Ampicillin
- ☐ D   Loperamide
- ☐ E   Intravenous fluids

Case 42

A 22-year-old man presents with a fever and abdominal pain. He is a medical student who has been on a 10-week elective to Kenya and Sudan. He took malarial prophylaxis and continued this as prescribed on his return to the UK 4 weeks ago.

On examination: temperature is 39.1°C, heart rate 110 bpm, blood pressure 115/60 mmHg, chest is clear, abdomen has palpable 5-cm splenomegaly, no focal neurology in CNS.

Investigations:

Hb	10.0 g/dL
WCC	2.2×10^9/L
Neutrophils	1.6×10^9/L
Platelets	70×10^9/L
Sodium	145 mmol/L
Potassium	5.0 mmol/L
Urea	6.8 mmol/L
Creatinine	90 μmol/L
Bilirubin	14 μmol/L
AST	125 U/L
ALP	50 U/L
Albumin	31 U/L
Urine	negative

1   What is the best investigation to confirm the diagnosis?

☐ A   CT abdomen
☐ B   Bone marrow aspirate
☐ C   Splenic aspirate
☐ D   Laparotomy
☐ E   Blood cultures

Case 43

An 18-year-old student presents with a 4-day history of fever, headache, sore throat, hoarse voice, and a non-productive cough.

On examination: temperature is 38.9°C, heart rate 100 bpm regular, blood pressure 110/70 mmHg, respiratory rate 24 breaths/min. Chest – scattered coarse crepitations throughout the chest, no focal clinical consolidation. You notice some erythematous lesions on his lower legs.

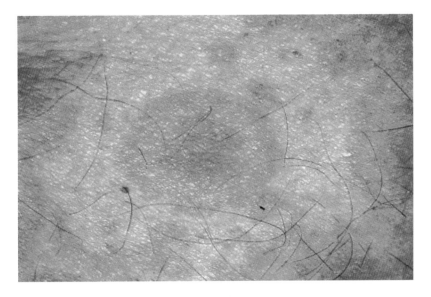

Investigations:

Hb	12.3 g/dL
WCC	8.0 × 10⁹/L
Neutrophils	6.6 × 10⁹/L
Platelets	200 × 10⁹/L
Sodium	139 mmol/L
Potassium	4.0 mmol/L
Urea	4.8 mmol/L
Creatinine	70 μmol/L
Bilirubin	8 μmol/L
AST	13 U/L
ALP	28 U/L
Albumin	42 U/L
CRP	60 mg/L

CXR – diffuse interstitial infiltrates in left lower lobe

1 **Which one of the following treatments should you prescribe?**

☐ A Oral prednisolone
☐ B Co-trimoxazole
☐ C Amoxicillin
☐ D Erythromycin
☐ E Ciprofloxacin

Case 44

A 59-year-old man presents with lethargy, abdominal distension, bilateral ankle swelling. He has no past medical history of note. He does not drink alcohol. He has never injected drugs. He is married with two children.

On examination: temperature is 38°C, heart rate 88 bpm, blood pressure 170/100 mmHg, hearts sound are normal, and there are no murmurs; there is bilateral pitting ankle oedema, the chest is clear, and the abdomen is distended with no palpable organs, shifting dullness is found.

Urine dipstick

Protein	++++
Blood	++++

Investigations:

Hb	8.7 g/dL
WCC	6.0×10^9/L
Neutrophils	4.6×10^9/L
Platelets	140×10^9/L
Sodium	139 mmol/L
Potassium	4.0 mmol/L
Urea	15.8 mmol/L
Creatinine	260 µmol/L
Bilirubin	120 µmol/L
AST	50 U/L
ALP	280 U/L
Albumin	22 U/L
CRP	10 mg/L

Urine culture   no growth

1   What test will help you identify the underlying cause?

A   HIV antibody test
B   Blood cultures
C   ANCA
D   Liver biopsy
E   Cryoglobulins

Case 45

A 52-year-old man is brought into A&E with a 1-day history of fever, rigors, and confusion. He had been unwell for the previous 3 days with a mild headache, muscle aches, and a dry cough.

On examination: temperature is 39.3°C, GCS 14/15, heart rate 120 bpm, blood pressure 100/60 mmHg, SpO$_2$ 90% on room air. Chest examination reveals right basal crepitations, in the abdomen there is right upper quadrant tenderness. CNS examination reveals mild photophobia, there is no neck stiffness, and no focal neurology.

Urine

Protein	+
Blood	+++

Investigations:

Hb	12.3 g/dL
WCC	5.0 × 10^9/L
Neutrophils	3.8 × 10^9/L
Platelets	140 × 10^9/L
Sodium	125 mmol/L
Potassium	4.8 mmol/L
Urea	13.8 mmol/L
Creatinine	90 μmol/L
Bilirubin	110 μmol/L
AST	300 U/L
ALP	110 U/L
Albumin	32 U/L
CRP	160 mg/L

ABG – on room air
pH	7.37
PCO$_2$	4.2 kPa
PO$_2$	9.3 kPa

1   Which one of the following is the most likely organism?

- [ ] A *Haemophilus influenzae*
- [ ] B *Mycoplasma pneumoniae*
- [ ] C *Staphylococcus aureus*
- [ ] D *Legionella pneumophila*
- [ ] E *Pseudomomas aeruginosa*

2   Which one of the following treatments should you prescribe?

- [ ] A   Ciprofloxacin
- [ ] B   Amoxicillin
- [ ] C   Clarithromycin
- [ ] D   Flucloxacillin
- [ ] E   Vancomycin

Case 46

A 25-year-old woman presents with a 10-day history of fever, drenching night sweats, and a headache. She recently underwent deep cleaning dental work. No past medical history.

On examination: her temperature is 38.6°C, GCS 15/15, heart rate 100 bpm, blood pressure 90/60 mmHg, auscultation of the praecordium reveals a harsh pansystolic murmur at the apex. The chest is clear. In the abdomen the tip of the spleen is palpable. There is no photophobia, neck stiffness or focal neurology.

1 Which one of the following is the most likely organism?

- ☐ A *Enterococcus* sp.
- ☐ B *Staphylococcus aureus*
- ☐ C *Coxiella burnetii*
- ☐ D *Streptococcus viridans*
- ☐ E *Staphylococcus epidermidis*

Case 47

A 19-year-old gap year student attends with a fever, shortness of breath, and a rash on her lower legs. She has been travelling throughout the United States of America, and has just flown back. She visited New York City, Las Vegas, the Grand Canyon, the Mississippi delta and flew back from Denver, Colorado.

On examination she has a temperature of 38.2°C, is alert and orientated. The heart rate is 120 bpm, blood pressure 100/70 mmHg and the heart sounds are normal. In the chest there is scattered bilateral wheeze. In the abdomen there are no palpable organs. There is no photophobia neck stiffness or focal neurology. There are multiple hard, tender nodules on both shins.

Investigations:

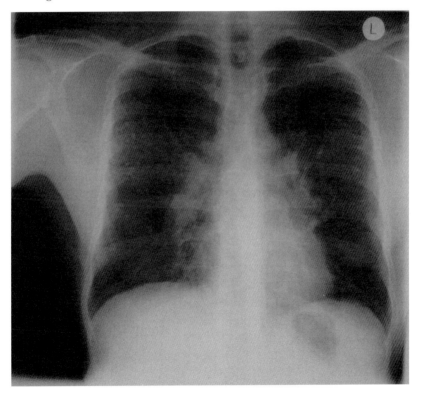

1   What treatment should you commence?

☐   A   Itraconazole
☐   B   Erythromycin
☐   C   Amoxicillin
☐   D   Prednisolone
☐   E   Low molecular weight heparin

Case 48

A 31-year-old intravenous drug user was diagnosed with chronic hepatitis C infection 10 months ago. He has read that there is a treatment of PEG-IFN and ribavirin that can be used to treat him and wants to try it.

Investigations:

Hb	11.5 g/dL
WCC	6.0×10^9/L
Neutrophils	4.8×10^9/L
Platelets	300×10^9/L
Sodium	145 mmol/L
Potassium	4.3 mmol/L
Urea	3.8 mmol/L
Creatinine	60 µmol/L
Bilirubin	11 µmol/L
AST	30 U/L
ALP	80 U/L
Albumin	32 U/L

Genotype	type 2
HCV viral load	800,000 copies /mL
α-FP	3 kU/L

1   Which factor predicts a better treatment outcome – sustained viral response (SVR) better than the others?

☐   A   Normal liver function tests
☐   B   Fibrosis score
☐   C   High HCV viral load
☐   D   Genotype 2
☐   E   Genotype 1

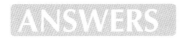

ANSWERS

Chapter One   Answers

HIV AND GENITOURINARY MEDICINE

Case 1

1   **C**   *Pneumocystis jiroveci** pneumonia (PCP) (formerly known as *Pneumocystis carinii* pneumonia)

2   **C**   Exercise oximetry
      G   Induced sputum

Pneumocystis jiroveci is the causative agent of PCP (qv *Book 1 – Respiratory* Q12 pp. 72, 133). This may be the de novo presentation of advanced immunosuppression and is classically characterised by the following symptoms:

- Dry non-productive cough
- Progress breathlessness on minimal exertion
- Fever
- Night sweats
- Weight loss.

The pertinent investigations are, ABG on room air, CXR (which may be normal in up to 50% of cases), exercise oximetry and induced sputum (in which to identify cysts or trophozoites using fluorescent monoclonal antibodies). If the CXR is normal, a high-resolution CT may help to identify 'ground-glass' shadowing. If induced sputum is negative or the procedure is not well tolerated then a bronchoscopy with bronchoalveolar lavage (BAL) can be performed and the BAL can be sent for immunofluoresence studies; careful timing of bronchoscopy is required particularly if the patient is hypoxic.

In this CXR note the classic features associated with PCP:

- Bilateral hilar lymphadenopathy
- Bilateral diffuse interstitial infiltrates
- Relative sparing of the apices
- Absence of pleural effusion and lobar consolidation.

Exercise oximetry is an easy method to test for desaturation

- Six-minute test on an exercise bike or treadmill
- A positive test is the occurrence of desaturation to ≤90% , or >5% drop from baseline
- It is a useful positive predictor of PCP in patients with HIV, but becomes less useful with subsequent episodes of PCP.

Treatment of PCP:

- First-line treatment – co-trimoxazole (Septrin®) iv or high-dose oral
- Alternatives
  clindamycin + primaquine
  dapsone + trimethoprim
  intravenous pentamidine
  atovaquone.
- Severity assessment by ABG: patients with
  $PO_2 > 10$ kPa – may be considered for outpatient treatment
  $PO_2 < 10$ kPa (or with a normal oxygen tension but an increased respiratory rate) – will probably require admission and require supplemental oxygen
  $PO_2 < 8.0$ kPa – the use of steroids is indicated to reduce the risk of developing ARDS and respiratory failure
- On proving the diagnosis of PCP, it is vital to elicit the cause of immunosuppression – here chronic HIV infection; all clinicians should be able to counsel and arrange for an HIV test.

* *Pneumocystis jiroveci* Frenkel 1999 is present in humans, *Pneumocystis carinii* only in rats, for clarity in the literature the abbreviation PCP has been kept.

Case 2

1   **D**   Kaposi's sarcoma

2   **B**   Human herpes virus 8

Kaposi's sarcoma (KS) is caused by human herpes virus 8 (HHV8); it is characterised by purple to brown-black violaceous lesions that can appear as macules, patches, nodules or papules. They are not painful or itchy. The lesion can affect one or more of the following organs: skin, lungs, GI tract (mouth to anus).

KS is associated with the following groups of patients:

- AIDS-related KS – severe immunosuppression
- Immunocompromised KS – post transplantation
- Classic KS – elderly Mediterranean men – usually on the lower legs
- Endemic KS – endemic form in Africa.

Diagnosis – KS has a characteristic appearance on histology with the presence of spindle cell proliferation.

Treatment of KS – there is no definitive treatment although foscarnet, cidofovir and ganciclovir have anti-HHV8 activity.

Local injection of cutaneous lesions with vinblastine can help reduce the lesion, but is not practical if numerous lesions are present. Systemic chemotherapy with liposomal anthracyclines shows good results with a good side-effect profile.

The differential diagnosis of KS includes:

- Cutaneous bacillary angiomatosis – associated with infection by *Bartonella* sp (*B. henselae* or *B. quintana*). Lesions are often papular and red with a smooth or eroded surface, the papules may enlarge to form large pedunculated lesions, they may be solitary or multiple, subcutaneous nodules can also occur. Treatment is with erythromycin or doxycycline.
- Pyogenic granulomas – (syn. granuloma telangiectaticum, pregnancy tumour), common benign vascular lesion of the skin and mucosa of unknown aetiology occurring most commonly in children, pregnant women and in those taking the combined oral contraceptive, indinavir or retinoic acid derivatives.

Fixed drug eruptions are discussed in *Book 2* – pp 148, 149.

Case 3

1   **E**   Keratoderma blennorrhagica

2   **C**   *Salmonella*

Keratoderma blennorrhagica is characterised by a pustular hyperkeratotic eruption on the soles of both feet in association with reactive arthritis (cf *Book 3* – Rheumatology Q10, 14, 15). The rash can also affect the palms, scrotum, trunk and scalp.

Reactive arthritis can be considered as a post-infectious arthritis, so:

- Post-viral arthritis, eg parvovirus
- Post-streptococcal arthritis
  Rheumatic fever
  Arthritis
- Post-*Neisseria* arthritis (cf *Book 3* – Rheumatology Q10, pp 93, 158)
- Lyme disease
- Whipple disease
- Reactive arthritis.

Reactive arthritis is one of the seronegative spondylarthropathies, (also including ankylosing spondylitis, psoriatic arthropathy, inflammatory-disease-associated arthritis and undifferentiated spondylarthropathy). They are associated with HLA B27, which is present particularly in those with severe disease.

Reiter's syndrome is a particular clinical syndrome and is sometimes used synonymously with reactive arthritis. Its particular features are however:

- Conjunctivitis
- Urethritis
- Arthritis.

Infectious agents associated with triggering reactive arthritis are enteric or urogenital infections listed below – they may be isolated before or after the diagnosis of the condition.

- *Chlamydia trachomatis*
- *Yersinia, Shigella flexneri, Salmonella, Campylobacter*
- *Streptococcus viridans*
- *Mycoplasma pneumoniae.*

If an infective agent is not identified and there are no features to point towards another specific spondylarthropathy then the term 'undifferentiated spondylarthropathy' may be used.

Other extra-articular features associated with the seronegative spondlyarthropathies (and their specific associations) are:

- Eyes
  Conjunctivitis
  Uveitis (ankylosing spondylitis and inflammatory bowel disease)
- Skin and mucous membranes
  Oral ulceration
  Circinate balanitis (Reiter's/reactive)
  Keratoderma blennorrhagica (psoriasis)
  Nail dystrophy (psoriasis)
  Erythema nodosum (inflammatory bowel disease)
- Cardiac
  Aortitis (ankylosing spondylitis)
  Conduction defects

Case 4

1   **D**   HIV viral load

This man has symptoms of primary HIV infection, also known as HIV seroconversion illness. A maculopapular rash is a non-specific sign present in many acute viral and bacterial illnesses. However, several clinical signs are more frequently seen with primary HIV infection as listed below:

Symptoms	Frequency
Fever (mean >38°C)	>80%
Arthralgia/myalgia	40–80%
Rash	
Night sweats	
Lymphadenopathy	
Sore throat	
Fatigue	
Oral +/– Genital ulcers	10–40%
>2.5-kg weight loss	
Nausea/D+V	

Certain blood results should raise the suspicion of HIV infection – leukopenia and thrombocytopenia can occur in seroconversion. In chronic HIV infection look out for anaemia, leukopenia, thrombocytopenia and a raised globulin level.

Remember the window period

- HIV antibody tests can be negative for up to 3 months after exposure
- If clinically suspicious, then can order:

P24 antigen test:	80% sensitivity, 99% specificity
HIV RNA branch DNA test:	100% sensitivity, 95% specificity
HIV RNA PCR test:	100% sensitivity, 97% specificity.

Identification of active HIV RNA replication is the gold standard for confirming the diagnosis of primary HIV infection – this is the HIV viral load test.

The levels are extremely high – often over a 100,000 copies/mL.

False-positive rate is approximately 3–5% with these tests – often seen when the result is <5000 copies/mL.

In this case the patient has a viral load of >500,000 copies/mL, his P24 antigen subsequently became positive, then the antibody test.

Case 5

1   **E**   Combination antiretroviral therapy

Cryptosporidium parvum is a protozoan parasite and a leading cause of infectious diarrhoea in humans and cattle. Transmission occurs through animal-to-human or human-to-human contact, by recreational exposure to contaminated water or land, or by consumption of contaminated water and food.

The most frequent symptom is watery diarrhoea, which can range from mild to severe.

Severe and persistent infection often occurs in immunocompromised patients.

Treatment of cryptosporidium related diarrhoea:

- There is no effective antimicrobial agent
- Combination antiretroviral therapy is required to restore immune function and allow for cell-mediated immune responses to resolve the infection
- Anti-diarrhoeal agents such as loperamide and codeine phosphate provide symptomatic relief
- Important to adhere to food and water hygiene to avoid re-infection.

Case 6

1   **D**   Ganciclovir iv

2   **A**   Colonoscopy

This man has acute cytomegalovirus (CMV) retinitis until proven otherwise which is sight-threatening because of the proximity of the lesion to the macula. The classic appearance of CMV retinitis is the 'cheese and tomato pizza pie' appearance.

Symptoms of CMV retinitis:

- Asymptomatic – found on routine screening (all patients with CD4 count <100 cells)
- Blurred vision
- Pyrexia of unknown origin.

It is likely this patient has disseminated CMV infection

- CMV colitis – fever, pain on passing stool
- CMV cholangitis – right upper quadrant pain, tenderness, fever and vast elevation of ALP.

Diagnosis:

- Urgent referral to Ophthalmology
- CMV IgM – acute infection
- CMV IgG – latent infection (consider reactivation)
- CMV DEAFF test – is a rapid culture test which is highly specific but with poorer sensitivity than PCR
- Serum CMV PCR – is highly sensitive but not specific for active infection
- Colonoscopy – colonic ulceration, biopsy shows CMV inclusion bodies (Owl's eyes)
- Liver biopsy – CMV inclusion bodies.

Treatment for CMV retinitis/colitis/cholangitis

Four antiviral agents have activity against CMV

- Ganciclovir – iv, oral, ocular implant – first-line therapy
- Valganciclovir – oral
- Foscarnet – iv
- Cidofovir – iv.

Case 7

1   A   CSF India ink stain

This patient has a diagnosis of cryptococcal meningitis, caused by the encapsulated fungus *Cryptococcus neoformans*, which is an AIDS-defining illness. The reservoir for *Cryptococcus* is soil infested with pigeon droppings or eucalyptus trees. The classical symptoms on presentation are:

- Headache
- Fever
- Meningism
- Personality change.

Investigation of cryptococcal meningitis:

- Serum cryptococcal antigen test – CRAG
    Titres may reach up to 1 : 2,000,000
    Negative serum CRAG excludes cryptococcal disease
- Lumbar puncture
    Measure the opening pressure – if pressure >20 cmH$_2$O one needs to drain off the CSF until pressure is down to 20 cm and consider shunting (an alternative to daily lumbar puncture)
    Most patients who die during initial treatment have raised intracranial pressure
    India ink stain – demonstrates encapsulated yeast
    CSF CRAG – positive result equates to a diagnosis of cryptococcal meningitis.

Poor prognostic indicators:

- High initial CSF opening pressure
- Decreased level of consciousness
- High cryptococcal antigen titre
- Low CSF white cell count
- Low CSF glucose.

Treatment of cryptococcal meningitis:

- First-line – iv amphotericin B – liposomal amphotericin is available if there is renal impairment

- Second-line – iv fluconazole – high dose oral administration can be used in mild cases.

Duration of treatment:

- Initial therapy is for 2 weeks in responders
- Secondary prophylaxis is continued lifelong, unless there is evidence of immune restoration (CD_4 >200 cells/mm^3 for 6 months) with negative serum cryptococcal antigen test.

Complications:

- Obstructive hydrocephalus
- Amphotericin B is nephrotoxic.

Other CSF stains and their uses:

- CSF VDRL – to diagnose neurosyphilis – there are no signs of tabes dorsalis in this patient
- CSF PCR – to diagnose viral encephalopathies
- CSF silver stain – an old-fashioned test to stain for oligoclonal bands in multiple sclerosis
- CSF Ziehl–Neelsen stain – to stain for *Mycobacteria tuberculosis*, the CSF protein + glucose values could point towards *M. tuberculosis*, but the lack of CT findings and the minimally raised CSF WCC count make this unlikely.

Case 8

1   **B**   Sulphadiazine and pyrimethamine

This patient has cerebral toxoplasmosis caused by *Toxoplasma gondii*, an obligate intracellular protozoa. The risk of developing cerebral toxoplasmosis with a CD4 count <100 cells/mm^3 is high.

The differential diagnosis of this case includes:

- Cerebral toxoplasmosis
- Bacterial brain abscesses – treat with broad spectrum antifungals
- Fungal brain abscesses due to cryptococcosis – treat with amphotericin B
- Tuberculomas – treat with anti-TB medication
- Malignant glioma – treat with cranial irradiation + cisplatin-based chemotherapy.

However, multiple ring-enhancing lesions with the predilection for the basal ganglia make cerebral toxoplasmosis the most likely diagnosis.

Clinical signs include:

- Fever
- Headache

- Neurological deficits
- Seizures
- Altered mental status.

Diagnosis of cerebral toxoplasmosis:

- Serological:
    Negative serology (<1 : 16) makes toxoplasmosis unlikely (<10%)
    Raised toxoplasma titres (>1 : 16) or positive toxoplasma IgM are not diagnostic of acute infection but indicate a potential for reactivation
- CT or MRI brain scan
    Usually reveals characteristic multiple ring-enhancing lesions – MRI is more sensitive
    Toxoplasmosis frequently affects the basal ganglia
- Lumbar puncture
    Often not performed because of mass lesions
    If performed, results are often normal, although raised protein is not uncommon.

Diagnosis is often retrospective; empirical treatment for cerebral toxoplasmosis is commenced and the patient is monitored for radiological and clinical improvement in response to 2 weeks of treatment.

Treatment

- First-line – sulphadiazine and pyrimethamine with folinic acid
- Second line – clindamycin and pyrimethamine with folinic acid.

Duration of treatment

- Treatment is usually for a period of 8 weeks.

Case 9

1   **B**   Azithromycin

2   **D**   BCG

This man is severely immunocompromised and is at significant risk of developing an opportunistic illness in the next 6 months.

For individuals with low CD4 counts (below 200), medication can be prescribed to prevent specific opportunistic infections. Common drugs used include:

- Co-trimoxazole (Septrin®) – for PCP and toxoplasmosis
- Dapsone – for PCP
- Pentamidine nebuliser – for PCP
- Aciclovir – for recurrent herpes simplex infection

- Fluconazole – for *Cryptococcus neoformans*
- Azithromycin – for atypical mycobacterium (MAC – *Mycobacterium avium complex*) commenced if CD4 count <50 cells.

With respect to vaccinations all LIVE attenuated vaccines are best avoided in HIV-positive patients. These include:

- Rubella
- Measles
- Oral polio
- BCG
- Yellow fever.

Killed or recombinant vaccines are safe to be administered.

Case 10

1   B   Procaine penicillin

This woman has early infectious syphilis. Without adequate treatment there is a high risk of vertical transmission to the developing fetus at any stage during pregnancy both in utero or at delivery.

Treatments for syphilis in pregnancy:

- Procaine penicillin – im daily for 17 days is the gold standard for treatment of syphilis in pregnancy in an HIV-positive woman
- Benzathine penicillin – associated with treatment failure in HIV-positive pregnant women
- Doxycycline – FDA pregnancy category D, which means that it is known to be harmful to an unborn baby and will affect fetal tooth and bone development
- Erythromycin – inferior response compared to procaine penicillin.

Features of congenital syphilis

- Two-thirds of neonates are asymptomatic at birth
- Early congenital syphilis – age <2 years
    Snuffles – nasal discharge teaming with spirochaetes
    Mucous patches – condylomata lata
    Maculopapular rash
    Hepatosplenomegaly
    Osteochondritis
- Late congenital syphilis – age >2 years
    Frontal bossing
    Saddle nose
    Perforated palate

Hutchinson's triad – Hutchinson's incisors, interstitial keratitis, VIII nerve deafness.

See answer to Chapter 1, Case 12 pages 105–106.

Case 11

1   C   She should be offered post exposure prophylaxis for HIV infection.

Exposure to patient's body fluids, and therefore to the risk of transmission of blood-borne viruses, is a very real hazard for health-care workers (HCW). Transmission can occur through parenteral, mucous membrane, and non-intact skin exposures. The use of universal precautions when dealing with patients reduces risk but incidents will inevitably occur. The occupational health department or on-call microbiologist/virologist/infectious diseases physician should be contacted. Hospital or trust protocols and guidelines should then be followed, the risk of exposure should be assessed, and appropriate management should be instigated as soon as possible.

Risk assessment of exposure

	Type of exposure	Type of fluid/tissue
High risk	Percutaneous injury	Blood
	Mucous membrane exposure	Fluids containing blood
↓	Non-intact skin exposure	Potentially infectious fluid/tissue*
Low risk	Intact skin exposure	Urine

*Semen and vaginal secretions, cerebrospinal, synovial, pleural, peritoneal, pericardial, and amniotic fluids.

Risk of transmission of blood-borne virus following needlestick injury

Infection	Needlestick exposure transmission rate %
Hepatitis B (HBV)	
eAg-positive	20-40%
eAg-negative	1–6%
Hepatitis C (HCV)	1–10%
HIV	0.3%

The following are *suggestions* on management. Blood samples should be taken from the source patient (always with consent) and recipient HCW as soon as possible.

- **Hepatitis B** – HCW within the NHS will be vaccinated against hepatitis B. Previously vaccinated HCW who are known responders (adequate levels of sAb) do not require post-exposure prophylaxis (PEP). Prophylaxis of the non-vaccinated or non-responders depends on the source patient. If source patient is known sAg-positive, hepatitis B immune globulin (HBIG) should be administered (im injection) and a rapid course of hepatitis B vaccine should be commenced. A vaccinated HCW with unknown antibody response should have their serology checked immediately and be treated appropriately when known. HBIG is effective if given within 24 h. A second dose should be given at 1 month to non-responders. If the source patient status is unknown, assume sAg positivity if there is a high risk of BBV.

- **Hepatitis C** – The serostatus and/ or HCV PCR status of the source patient and HCW should be checked. There is no vaccination currently available and no standardised PEP. If the source is HCV-PCR-positive, the exposed HCW should have an HCV antibody, HCV PCR, and ALT performed at 3 and 6 months. Interferon-α and ribavirin have been used in early infection, resulting in high rates of clearance of virus.

- **HIV** – Although the risk of HIV transmission is low, this infection causes greatest concern to HCW. HIV seroconversion occurs following percutaneous exposure to HIV-infected blood in approximately 1 in 300 injuries. The risk is less than 1 in 1000 following mucous membrane exposure and nil with intact skin exposure. The risk of needle-stick transmission increases if the source patient has a high HIV viral load, if a large volume of blood is inoculated, if a hollow bore needle is used, or a deep injury is sustained. HIV transmission may be decreased using PEP. Four weeks of highly active antiretroviral therapy (HAART), usually consisting of three drugs, is given. Treatment should be given within 1 h of the exposure and should not be delayed while awaiting results if the injury is deemed high risk. PEP can always be stopped if the source is found to be HIV negative. However, the HCW must be aware that evidence is from animal and observational studies only and HAART has many side-effects and deaths have occurred during PEP treatment of HCW with HAART.

See: http://www.advisorybodies.doh.gov.uk; http://www.gmc-uk.org/guidance/library/serious_communicable_diseases.asp

Regarding our case, approximately 20% of those infected with hepatitis C clear the virus. They remain hepatitis C antibody positive but are HCV-PCR-negative (as in our case). This seropositivity does not confer immunity and re-infection can occur. Our active injecting drug user may therefore now be HCV-PCR-positive.

A high-risk injury has occurred from a high-risk patient with other previous BBV. HIV PEP should be offered to the HCW until HIV results are available.

Case 12

1   **B**   The results are consistent with secondary syphilis.

Elderly patients presenting with confusion should have treponemal serology performed as part of their laboratory work up. It is therefore helpful to be able to interpret these results.

The stages of syphilis are:

- Primary syphilis – a painless ulcer, the primary chancre, develops at the site of treponemal invasion, 10–90 days (mean 21 days) after contact. One sees localised lymphadenopathy
- Secondary syphilis – occurs 8 weeks later. The patient develops fever, headache, and lethargy. A macular, then papular, rash develops on trunk, palms, soles, and flexural surfaces which may last for 3 months. Half of patients develop generalised lymphadenopathy
- Latent syphilis – *T. pallidum* persists in the body without causing symptoms or signs. This is divided into:
  Early latent – when infection has occurred in the previous 12 months. The patient remains infectious
  Late latent – when infection has occurred > 12 months ago. The patient is non-infectious but maternal to foetal transfer can occur.
- Late or tertiary syphilis. A progressive inflammatory disease that can affect almost any organ, hence 'the great mimic'.
  Neurosyphilis can occur at any time (meningovascular syphilis, paretic syphilis, and tabes dorsalis).
  Other features manifest over the next 15–30 years.
    Gummata form in the skin or within visceral organs, eg liver, bone, CNS.
    Cardiovascular syphilis usually involves the aorta. Scarring wakens the aortic walls, leading to aneurysm formation and aortic valve incompetence.

The diagnosis can be made by observing spirochaetes in genital ulcer specimens under dark-field microscopy (normal oral flora includes other non-pathological treponemes); however, serology remains most important in diagnosis.

The immune response to syphilis involves the production of non-specific antibodies (cardiolipin or lipoidal antibody) and specific treponemal antibodies. Non-treponemal tests detect non-specific treponemal antibody, eg Venereal Diseases Research Laboratory (VDRL), Rapid Plasma Reagin (RPR). False positive results can occur in a wide range of conditions eg pregnancy, viral infections, connective tissue diseases, and their levels fall in late disease. However they are valuable for monitoring response to treatment and detecting relapse or re-infection. Treponemal tests detect specific treponemal antibody, eg *T. pallidum* haemagglutination assay (TPHA), *T. pallidum* particle agglutination (TPPA), enzyme immunoassay (EIA) tests, and the fluorescent treponemal antibody-absorbed test (FTA-abs). These tests remain positive for life.

	VDRL	EIA IgM	EIA IgG	TPPA/TPHA
Primary	+/-	+/-	+/-	+/-
Secondary	+	+/-	+	+
Early latent	+/-	-	+	+
Late latent	-	-	+	+
Treated	-	-	+	+

Non-venereal (endemic) treponemal infections have identical serological responses.

- Bejel (*T. pallidum* subsp. *endemicum*) – causes endemic syphilis in hot, dry, climates. Causes a primary chancre, chronic cases develop destructive bone and cartilage lesions
- Pinta (*T. pallidum* subsp. *carateum*) – only occurs in Central and South America and affects only the skin
- Yaws (*T. pallidum* subsp. *pertenue*) – remains endemic in many tropical countries. It is spread by direct skin contact, causing lesions in children. It persists as a chronic relapsing illness; 10% develop CNS and bone lesions after 10–20 years.

See answer to Chapter 1, Case 10 page 102.

Chapter Two   Answers

INFECTIOUS DISEASES

Case 1

1 **F** Bronchoalveolar lavage
   J High resolution CT scan of chest

2 **D** Sarcoidosis

This lady has erythema nodosum, bilateral hilar lymphadenopathy, constitutional symptoms, high serum calcium, and lymphopenia. The differential diagnosis is between sarcoidosis and tuberculosis. Her background suggests TB but the hypercalcaemia strongly favours sarcoidosis. Patients with TB, especially females and those from the Indian sub-continent, often have hypocalcaemia. (cf *Book 1* – Respiratory Question 6; *Book 2* – Dermatology Question 1 and *Book 3* – Haematology Question 9)

In the absence of a useful single test, the diagnosis of sarcoidosis relies on:

- A typical clinico-radiological presentation
- Histopathological evidence, eg demonstration of non-caseating granulomas
- Exclusion of other causes.

A bronchoalveolar lavage will be the most discriminant investigation. Microscopy using Ziehl–Neelsen stain would show the presence or absence of acid–alcohol-fast bacteria (AAFB). Diagnostic microscopy has a sensitivity of 50–90% depending on clinical presentation. In the absence of AAFB, subsequent mycobacterial culture will be positive in >30% of cases of TB. White cell differentials from BAL fluid are of diagnostic value. Lymphocytes predominate in sarcoid and studies on lymphocyte subpopulations in BAL are helpful. A CD4 : CD8 ratio > 3.5 has a sensitivity of 53%, a specificity of 94%, a positive predictive value of 76%, and a negative predictive value of 85%.[1] Transbronchial biopsy may be performed at the same time and may reveal non-caseating granulomas in 40–90% of cases of saroid. A high-resolution CT (HRCT) will further resolve the nature of the lung pathology and will be useful in staging the disease.

Typical findings on HRCT include:

- Widespread small nodules with a bronchovascular and subpleural distribution
- Thickened interlobular septae

- Architectural distortion
- Conglomerate masses.

Serum angiotensin-converting enzyme (ACE) is elevated in many conditions, eg other granulomatous diseases (including TB and Langerhans cell histiocytosis – qv *Book 3* – Endocrine Question 8) and hyperthyroidism. ACE may be used in the monitoring of disease activity or response to treatment. An autoantibody screen may yield false-positive antinuclear antibodies (ANA), and elevated rheumatoid factor (RF) in sarcoidosis. An elevated ESR is non-specific. A 24-h urinary calcium will show hypercalciuria (seen in >40% patients with sarcoid); however, we know already that this patient has hypercalcaemia. The patient has no productive cough therefore there is no sputum for microscopy and culture.

The Mantoux test will be difficult to interpret. A strongly positive test may be seen in an Indian-born doctor without active TB, whereas sarcoidosis can produce anergy and an absent reaction. Skin biopsy of erythema nodosum will only show a paniculitis and give no clue to the cause. An HIV-antibody test, while recommended, will not add to the diagnosis.

Case 2

1   **B**   *Escherichia coli*
     F   *Campylobacter jejuni*
     G   *Salmonella*

This elderly diabetic lady has a severe diarrhoeal illness characterised by acute renal failure, thrombocytopenia, and anaemia. There is a likely source and incubation period (the meat pie 24–36 hours before symptom onset) but remember that outbreaks of viral gastroenteritis, especially norovirus (previously Norwalk virus), occur at institutions such as hospitals, care homes, and schools.

Incubation periods for enteric pathogens:

Organism	Incubation	Organism	Incubation
Bacillus cereus	1–6 hours	*Vibrio parahaemolyticus*	24–72 hours
Staphylococcus aureus	2–7 hours	*Shigella* spp.	12–96 hours
Clostridium perfringens	8–12 hours	*E. coli* 0157	1–4 days
Salmonella spp.	8–48 hours	*Vibrio cholerae*	1–5 days
E. coli (enterotoxic)	12–72 hours	*Campylobacter jejuni*	1–10 days
Viral gastroenteritis eg norovirus, rotavirus	1–3 days	*Cryptosporidium parvum*	7–14 days
		Entamoeba histolytica	~14–28 days

The secretory and toxin-mediated diarrhoeas (those with short incubation periods) and viral gastroenteritis tend not to cause non-bloody diarrhoea. *Vibrio parahaemolyticus* is usually transmitted from shellfish. There is nothing in the history suggesting recent admission to hospital or antibiotic use, making *Clostridium difficile* unlikely; it can be sporadic but usually occurs 5–10 days following antibiotics.

2   **B**   An urgent blood film should be performed

She does not have diabetic ketoacidosis. She is a tablet-controlled type 2 diabetic and her bicarbonate is 19 mmol/L. Ketonuria reflects poor food intake. The absence of neutrophilia and fever is well recognised in the elderly. Her diuretics should be discontinued. 'Food poisoning' is a notifiable illness to the Health Protection Agency (HPA). A microbiological cause is identified in approximately 50% of cases only. As well as completing a notification form, this particular case must be discussed with a public health doctor as soon as possible.

3   **B**   *Escherichia coli*

This lady has HUS as a result of *E. coli* 0157 (an enterohaemorrhagic or verocytotoxic *E. coli*). A blood film will show red cell fragmentation. Well-publicised outbreaks have occurred in recent years, usually in association with undercooked beef, dairy produce, and cold meats. The organism produces a verotoxin, resulting in invasive diarrhoea and vascular endothelial damage in the GI system, kidney, and CNS. A spectrum of illness between HUS and TTP may be seen (qv *Book 3* – Haematology Question 15). Elderly patients often develop neurological symptoms.

Treatment is usually supportive. The use of antibiotics is controversial. In large outbreaks antibiotics have been shown to increase mortality in the elderly.

(cf *Book 2* – Gastroenterology Question 17)

Case 3

1   **E**   Antibiotic treatment should be given before the lumbar puncture

2   **A**   iv aciclovir and iv cefotaxime

3   **B**   Herpes simplex 2 (HSV-2)

This woman has an encephalitic illness following a possible sexually transmitted infection. She has meningism and a lymphocytic CSF. The most common cause of sporadic encephalitis is herpes simplex virus type 1.

Herpes simplex virus type 1 (HSV-1) or human herpes virus 1 (HHV-1) usually causes oral lesions and HHV-2/HSV-2 causes genital lesions, but occasionally the converse is true. Recurrences can occur throughout the patient's lifetime because herpes viruses (also VZV, EBV) remain dormant in the nervous system after primary infection.

HSV encephalitis usually occurs as a reactivation of infection but may also occur with the primary illness (the case in the question may allude to either). The virus has a predilection for the temporal lobes, and affects this in around two thirds of patients. HSV-1 is a more common cause of encephalitis in adults (it accounts for 95% of all fatal cases of sporadic encephalitis) than HSV-2, the latter usually causes meningitis.

Clinical presentation

- Following a short prodrome of fever, lethargy, and headache, lasting 24–72 h, the illness progresses with signs of severe CNS dysfunction
- Patients develop delirium, fluctuating level of consciousness, seizures, aphasia, and other focal deficits, eg cranial nerve lesions and hemiparesis
- This progresses to coma and death in 60–80% of untreated patients within 7–14 days

Investigations

- CSF
    PCR – the most sensitive and specific test
        following DNA amplification a Southern blot identifies the characteristic herpes simplex banding. The results are positive early in the disease and the test produces a result quickly – it is now considered the gold standard for the diagnosis of encephalitis due to either HSV-1 or HSV-2
            it remains positive for 3–5 days after definitive treatment has been commenced
    culture – one cannot routinely culture virus from the CSF or blood
    M,C&S and biochemistry – aseptic CSF with a lymphocytosis and an elevated protein may support the diagnosis
- EEG – this may show abnormalities in up to 80%. Diffuse slowing and focal temporal lobe abnormalities eg periodic spike and slow-wave patterns can support the diagnosis but are non-specific. It can be normal for the first 48 h.
- Brain biopsy – insensitive and can result in serious complications (oedema and haemorrhage)
- MRI – more sensitive than CT. CT may remain normal for 3–4 days. MRI may demonstrate hypo-dense areas in the temporal lobes to support the diagnosis

Treatment

- Aciclovir 10 mg/kg 8-hourly iv should be commenced in all patients where a diagnosis of HSV encephalitis is considered. It can reduce mortality to less than 25%. It should be continued for 14–21 days monitor for crystalluria and renal toxicity

A CT scan must be performed before lumbar puncture in patients with focal neurological signs, seizures, or a change in level of consciousness. The CSF result suggests viral meningitis but this patient is very unwell and until bacterial meningitis is excluded it must be covered with appropriate antibiotics. Administer antibiotics urgently in all patients with suspected meningoencephalitis. Never defer until after lumbar puncture.

Purpura is a feature of meningococcaemia (and DIC), not meningitis per se. Of course meningococcaemia can be a consequence of meningeal infection but the absence of a rash is simply non-contributory. Drowsiness can be a feature of bilateral cortical disease as well as functional or structural impairment of the reticular activating system (RAS), as such in this case there is nothing to indicate involvement of the RAS. The framing of the question may lead one to consider listeria meningitis – but this occurs at the extremes of age and in the immunocompromised. It is the most common organism in meningitis; in rhomboencephalitis is more common eg cranial nerve palsies, as are seizures. CSF may be lymphocytic and is often aseptic, the glucose is low in c. 50% and the protein high mimicking TB or fungal infection; Gram positive bacilli are seen in 10–40% of cases, however if organisms are seen they can be Gram variable and look like diplococci or diphtheroids; treatment is by addition of ampicillin to the regime until the diagnosis is made by culture of the CSF and/or blood. cf. Book 2 Neurology Case 17. Regarding HIV seroconversion cf. Chapter 1 Case 6.

Case 4

This patient is returning from rural Africa with a febrile illness with a possible rash, bruising, and a sore throat. While malaria is top of the differential diagnosis, the possibility of a viral haemorrhagic fever has to be considered. While there have been no cases of Ebola or Marburg virus infection imported into the UK, with the world's increasingly mobile population a case might one day present to your hospital. Cases of yellow fever, Lassa fever, and dengue haemorrhagic fever have been seen.

If this possibility is considered then the patient must be placed in isolation, nursed with gowns/gloves/masks, and discussed as soon as possible with the local infectious diseases specialist (they will in turn contact specialists in Newcastle or Coppetts Wood if necessary, the UK's high-security isolation facilities). No samples should be taken until a risk assessment has been made. See http://www.hpa.org.uk.

1   **E**   Yellow fever is an unlikely differential diagnosis

The yellow fever vaccine is almost 100% effective and immunity persists for at least 10 years (hence yellow fever certificates are valid for 10 years). Hence yellow fever is unlikely.

2   **B**   Treatment may be complicated by severe hypoglycaemia
     G   The infection can be transmitted via needlestick injury
     I   He has severe falciparium malaria

The patient has severe falciparum malaria with haemolytic anaemia, renal impairment, and DIC. Non-falciparum malaria rarely causes a parasitaemia above 1% and complications are unusual. The film shows red cells containing more then one 'ring-form', also typical of falciparum malaria.

Indicators of severe falciparum malaria are:

parasitaemia of ≥2% and/or one or more of the following complications:

- Cerebral malaria
    Disturbed level of consciousness
    Coma
    Seizures
    Focal signs
- Hypoglycaemia
- Renal impairment – ATN from hypovolaemia
- Pulmonary oedema
- Acute respiratory distress syndrome
- Haemolytic anaemia – may result in haemoglobinuria 'blackwater fever' as illustrated in the picture
- DIC
- Septic shock – because of Gram-negative sepsis, syn. 'algid malaria'

Investigations in severe malaria

- FBC – anaemia, leucopaenia or pancytopaenia. Thrombocytopaenia is a very useful clue to *P. falciparum*
- Blood film – repeat thick films to identify parasites and thin films to quantify the parasataemia. A *skilled* microscopist looking at films is still the gold standard
- Malaria antigen – approaches the sensitivity of a *skilled* microscopist
- U&E – renal impairment or failure

- LFT – hyperbilirubinaemia which reflects the degree of haemolysis and transaminitis
- CT – to exclude other pathology if cerebral malaria is suspected

Treatment:

- iv quinine – the drug of choice and acceptable even with G6PD deficiency in acute malaria
    Beware of conduction disturbances and hypoglycaemia
    Oral quinine can be use in uncomplicated falciparum malaria (alternatives are artemether, mefloquine, malarone)
    Following quinine, doxycycline is given to eradicate the remaining asexual stages of the parasite
    An alternative is fansidar (pyrimethamine/sulphadoxine) but this has significant side-effects and resistance is recognised
    Primaquine is used to kill liver hypnozoites of *Plasmodium ovale* and *P. vivax* after treatment with chloroquine, It is not used in *P. falciparum* infection

(qv *Book 3* – Haematology Question 11)

Case 5

1 **D** Tuberculous meningitis (TBM)

2 **A** An HIV antibody test can be performed without his consent
    D He should be commenced on anti-epileptic medication
    F An MRI scan will further aid diagnosis

Most UK cases of TB are seen in immigrants, especially economic or political refugees. There is a 5–10% lifetime risk of active TB following primary pulmonary tuberculosis. Risk increases with HIV infection, malnutrition, alcoholism, diabetes mellitus, corticosteroid use and malignancy.

TBM occurs when bacilli seed to the CNS, forming subependymal foci of tubercles. Tubercles rupturing into the subarachnoid space cause meningitis. Those deeper in the brain or spinal cord parenchyma may cause tuberculomas. Basal meningitis is typical, with inflammation, vasculitis, and thick exudates. Therefore, one commonly sees cranial nerves palsies (nerve VI most frequently, then III, IV, and VII) and obstructive hydrocephalus.

Differential diagnosis of a chronic meningitis illness:

Bacterial	Parasitic	Neoplastic
TBM	Cysticercosis	Lymphoma
Brain abscess	Toxoplasmosis	Metastases
Listeria meningitis	Trypanosomiasis	
Brucellosis		Inflammatory
Lyme disease	Viral	Sarcoidosis
Leptospirosis	Herpesviruses	Vasculitis
Syphilis	HIV-1	
Actinomycosis	HTLV-1	
Nocardiasis		
	Fungal	
	Cryptococcus	
	Histoplasmosis	

CSF examination should be performed in all cases of suspected TBM. Positive mycobacterial culture should be possible to achieve in up to 80% of TBM cases but takes over 2 weeks. PCR can give more rapid results. CT scan and MRI of the brain may reveal hydrocephalus, basilar meningeal thickening, infarcts, oedema and tuberculomas.

Treat with four anti-tuberculous drugs for at least 12 months. Even with treatment the mortality is as high as 15–30% in the UK. (cf *Book 2* – Endocrinology Question 16, 26, Gastroenterology Question 10, 16; *Book 3* – Rheumatology Case 11).

Regarding this case, an HIV antibody test can be performed without his consent. The GMC Guidelines on Communicable Diseases[2] state *'…you may test unconscious patients for serious communicable diseases, without their prior consent, where testing would be in their immediate clinical interests…'*; in this case it would be. The investigations and treatment of TB are free to all patients. He should be commenced on anti-epileptic medication as he has had two witnessed generalised seizures and is at risk of more. There is no role for iv mannitol at this time. A normal CXR does not exclude active pulmonary TB, but he is being ventilated on a closed circuit system and therefore does not require nursing in a side room.

Case 6

1   **B**   Jejunal biopsy
    C   String test
    G   Stool microscopy and culture

2   **E**   Ivermectin 200 µg/kg/day for 2 days

This patient has strongyloidiasis with possible hyperinfection. He is from an endemic area and consumes excess alcohol. He also has hyperglycaemia. His blood tests show a marked eosinophilia with evidence of malabsorption. The colonic biopsy results suggest a widespread inflammation involving both small and large bowel.

Strongyloides stercoralis infects more than 50 million people in the tropics and sub-tropics. Infection occurs after free-living filariform larvae penetrate the skin. Larval penetration and migration to the small bowel via the lungs can cause an acute illness with an itchy erythematous rash, pulmonary symptoms, eosinophilia, and diarrhoea. The adult worms produce eggs within the bowel which hatch before being released in faeces. Autoinfection by larvae via the colonic mucosa (hence colonic inflammation) or perianal skin, means that the parasite can persist 'indefinitely' within the host.

Chronic infections are asymptomatic in >50% and eosinophilia can be an incidental finding in some patients. Migrating larvae produce the pathognomic larva currens, a pruritic, creeping eruption affecting the trunk. Symptoms may resemble peptic ulcer disease, with diarrhoea and features of bowel obstruction if infection is heavy.

Hyperinfection occurs in patients with immunodeficiency, eg those taking steroids or immunosuppressants, those with malignancy, or with HTLV-1 infection, but is rare in HIV infection. Dissemination can occur to the lungs, CNS, liver, and kidneys. Mortality from hyperinfection is high – between 25 and 100%.

Diagnosis depends on identifying the larvae on microscopic examination of stool (direct or after culture) or samples obtained from small bowel, eg biopsy, duodenal aspirate, or string test. In the latter, a capsule attached to a length of string is swallowed. Later, when the capsule has passed into the small bowel, the string is withdrawn. Mucus and fluid on the string can then be observed on a microscope slide. Serological methods, eg ELISA, may be useful.

Treatment is with ivermectin. Thiabendazole is a useful but unpleasant alternative. Albendazole is less effective.

Other causes of small bowel malabsorption suggested in the answers include:

- Whipple's disease – a rare multisystem infection caused by *Tropheryma whipplei*, usually presenting with arthropathy and abdominal symptoms in middle-aged white men; it rarely causes eosinophilia, diagnosis is by small bowel biopsy (PAS-positive macrophages) and treatment is usually with ceftriaxone or meropenem.
- Giardiasis – can cause abdominal discomfort, diarrhoea, and excessive wind. One would not expect as severe an illness as this

gentleman has and colonic inflammation would be unusual. It is diagnosed using stool microscopy, duodenal or jejunal aspirate/biopsy, or the string test. Treatment is either metronidazole or a single dose of tinidazole 2 g. (cf *Book 2* – Gastroenterology Question 12)

Causes of eosinophilia

- Parasitic
  Ascaris (Löfflers syndrome)
  Helminths – *Strongyloides*, Schistosomiasis, *Trichinella*, Filarial, Onchocerciasis, Paragonimiasis
  Toxocara – visceral larva migrans
  Echinococcus granulosum
  Necator americanus, Ancylostoma duodenale – hookworm
- Fungal
  Coccidioidomycosis
  Aspergillus – ABPA
- Viral
  HIV
  HTLV-1
- Immunological
  Atopy – asthma, dermatitis, eczema, allergic rhinitis
  Sarcoidosis
  Polyarteritis nodosa
  Transplant rejection
  Drug induced
  Job's syndrome (hyper-IgE syndrome)
- Rheumatological
  Churg–Strauss syndrome
  Eosinophilic vasculitis
- Pulmonary
  ABPA
  Tropical pulmonary eosinophilia – filarial
  Eosinophilic pneumonia
  Neoplasia
- Haematological
  Hypereosinophilic syndromes – idiopathic
  Leukaemia
  Lymphoma
- Skin
  Atopy
  Urticaria
  Pemphigoid
- Endocrinological – Addison's disease

- Neoplastic
- Drugs
  - NSAIDs
  - GM-CSF (not G-CSF)
- Other – cholesterol emboli.

Case 7

1 **B** Chloroquine and proguanil

2 **C** Yellow fever

3 **E** *Schistosoma mansoni*

A young doctor returns from Africa with a febrile illness with a non-specific rash and few other clues except for the history of contact with fresh water (sailing).

Any of the prophylaxis regimens would be appropriate except for chloroquine and proguanil. While a detailed knowledge of anti-malarial prophylaxis would not be necessary for a candidate sitting MRCP, the knowledge that *Plasmodium falciparum* resistance to chloroquine is widespread, especially in sub-Saharan Africa, is expected. Doxycycline is taken daily but can cause a photosensitivity rash and GI upset. Mefloquine is taken weekly but can cause neuropsychiatric side-effects and GI upset. Maloprim, as a weekly dose, is effective but used infrequently in the UK. Malarone is usually well tolerated but is an expensive, daily tablet. Its advantage is that it can be taken from the day before travel until 1 week after return (other regimens are from 1 week before to 4 weeks after return).

The differential diagnosis list is very large and includes:

- Malaria – always the most important and will have to be excluded with three negative films and/or a malarial antigen test. The use of the correct prophylaxis and bite prevention methods only *reduces* the probability of infection.
- Enteric fever (usually *Salmonella typhi* or *S. paratyphi*) and dengue fever should be near the top of this differential diagnosis.
- Typhoid vaccination gives only partial immunity and dengue fever is spread by the day-biting *Aedes* mosquito and is therefore difficult to prevent.
- Yellow fever is most unlikely because vaccination (which the doctor will have received as it is a legal requirement to travel between most African countries) is >99% effective.

Katayama fever is the diagnosis in this case. At representation he has chronic schistosomiasis due to *Schistosoma mansoni* infection. Infection follows exposure to motile larvae in fresh water that have developed in an intermediate snail host. The larvae penetrate the skin, often causing a pruritic eruption, 'swimmers itch', before migrating to either the mesenteric (*S. mansoni, S. japonicum*) or vesical (*S. haematobium*) venules, where the adult flukes grow and produce eggs. During migration an immune-complex-like illness can develop, known as Katayama fever. Eggs are released into the colon or bladder and hatch in water when excreted in stool or urine; however, some are retained and cause inflammation of local structures leading to fibrosis and scarring of the colon and bladder. Late complications include portal hypertension and oesophageal varices, and carcinoma of the bladder. Migration to other sites can occur, eg lungs, CNS.

Diagnosis is by visualisation of the eggs in stool or urine (using concentration techniques). Serology is of use in diagnosing chronic disease in travellers but is often negative in acute disease. Treatment is with praziquantel in two or three divided doses.

Results of the stool sample:

- *Strongyloides stercoralis* larvae, not eggs, are seen in faeces.
- *Trichinella spiralis* larvae develop in muscle after ingestion of undercooked meat, its eggs are not seen in the faeces.
- *Ancylostoma duodenale* is a hookworm and causes iron deficiency anaemia.
- *Ascaris lumbricoides* is a roundworm and causes abdominal discomfort and occasionally intestinal obstruction.
- Both *Ancylostoma* and *Ascaris* are diagnosed by observing eggs in faeces.

Case 8

1 **C** Amoebic liver abscess (ALA)

2 **E** Amoebic serology
   G Aspiration of abscess

This young man returns from a holiday in the tropics with fever and a liver mass. His bloods indicate a chronic septic process and immunity to hepatitis B – antibodies to HBsAg (ie anti-HBsAb) imply vaccination (he is a medical student and has received immunisation).

The most likely diagnosis is ALA. This occurs following infection with *Entamoeba histolytica* by ingestion of cyst-contaminated water or food. The *Entamoeba* may invade the colonic epithelium (10% of infections) and spread to the liver (<1%) via the portal circulation. Here, *E. histolytica* causes apoptosis of hepatocytes and neutrophils, forming the characteristic 'anchovy paste' pus. ALA is more common in young adults, and males (10 : 1). The abscesses are often solitary and are most commonly within the right lobe. Abscesses will grow inexorably until rupture into the peritoneal, pleural, or pericardial cavities, or through the skin.

Diagnosis is made by US or CT, positive amoebic serology (indirect fluorescent antibody test, enzyme immunoassay), and an appropriate epidemiological history. Aspiration may be performed to exclude a PLA, but amoebal trophozoites are only seen in 15–20% of cases so its diagnostic value in ALA is limited. Notwithstanding this, the presence of an odourless, 'anchovy paste', sterile aspirate in the correct clinical setting suggests an ALA as opposed to thin, malodorous or frothy pus, which is more in keeping with PLA. Stool microscopy for amoebic cysts and trophozoites is of little value as asymptomatic carriage following travel is common, and a positive result is seen in 20% of ALA cases.

Treatment is with 10 days of oral metronidazole 800 mg tds followed by 10 days of either diloxanide furorate or paromamycin (luminal amoebicides). Aspiration may be performed in treatment failure or if rupture seems imminent.

PLA is less likely in this case. Clues to a PLA may lie within the history. The patient is often male, and in their fifth or sixth decade. There may be a source of infection, eg biliary sepsis, direct spread from contiguous infection, recent abdominal operation or instrumentation of the biliary tree, intravenous drug abuse, and recent venous canulation. Abscesses are often multiple. Causative organisms are usually related to the underlying pathology and often mixed, eg coliforms, *Enterococcus* spp., *Streptococcus* spp. (including *S. milleri*), and anaerobes. Abscesses can be visualised on US or CT scan but cannot be differentiated from ALA. Diagnosis is by culture of aspiration fluid and blood cultures. Treatment involves drainage – often percutaneous – and prolonged antibiotics.

Patients with hydatid disease (due to *Echinococcus granulosus*) usually present with pressure symptoms because of the cysts (liver 70%, lung 20%, spleen and peritoneal cavity). This occurs many months or years after infection and often the patient remains systemically well unless presenting with cyst rupture. Imaging may reveal calcification in 40% and/or daughter cysts (qv *Book 2* – Gastroenterology Question 23).

Brucellosis can rarely cause hepatic abscesses but there is nothing in the history to suggest this diagnosis except for foreign travel.

HCC arises in 60–90% of cases in a cirrhotic liver – most commonly worldwide as a result of chronic HBV infection, otherwise alcoholism or haemochromatosis are common causes; it may occur after a lag of 20–50 years from the primary liver injury. It is most commonly a solitary lesion, which enhances in the arterial phase of CT, α-FP is elevated in 80% of cases (qv *Book 2* – Gastroenterology Question 13).

Case 9

1   **D**   Mumps

This is a young student with a febrile illness characterised by tender facial swelling, lymphadenopathy, and pelvic pain. She is pyrexial with mild neck stiffness but no other signs of meningism.

Mumps is usually a self-limiting viral infection of childhood. After a febrile prodrome, most patients develop painful swelling of the salivary glands, usually parotids, unilateral or bilateral, which usually resolve after 7 days. Orchitis is a painful complication seen in 20–35% of adolescent males and can cause sterility. Women can develop oophoritis –as in our patient, but this very rarely causes sterility. Other complications include lymphocytic meningoencephalitis (rarely cranial nerve palsies and deafness), pancreatitis, myocarditis, and arthritis.

Pancreatitis can manifest with classical symptoms or can be asymptomatic with a hyperamylasaemia. An elevated serum amylase is often seen because of the release of salivary amylase – this can be differentiated from pancreatic amylase.

Diagnosis is often clinical but can be confirmed by mumps urinary antigen or serology. Infection results in lifelong immunity.

MMR (measles-mumps-rubella) vaccine should be given at 12–15 months of age. In 1998 The Lancet published a paper regarding a possible link between the combined MMR vaccination and the subsequent development of autism. This paper and the associated coverage resulted in a reduction in the uptake of childhood vaccinations, in particular MMR. Outbreaks of these infections have occurred and may continue to occur wherever the prevalence of unvaccinated individuals is high.

Incubation periods of childhood infections.

Virus	Transmission	Incubation (days)	Prodrome (days)
Mumps	Respiratory, droplets	12–25	2–3
Measles	Respiratory, droplets	7–18	2–4
Rubella	Respiratory, droplets	14–21	Child nil Adult 1–5
Chickenpox	Respiratory, droplets or direct contact	13–21	Mild variable
EBV	Saliva	30–50	Variable
Parvovirus B19	Respiratory, droplets or direct contact	2–5	2–5

Table (*continued*)

Virus	Infective from	Infective till
Mumps	1 week before parotitis	10 days after parotitis
Measles	Before symptoms	4 days after rash appears
Rubella	1 week before rash	4 days after rash appears.
Chickenpox	2 days before rash	Until lesions all scabbed
EBV	Unknown	Up to 18 months after symptoms resolve
Parvovirus B19	During prodrome, before rash	When rash appears

Case 10

1 **A** Malaria film
   B Blood cultures
   E Chest X-ray

This lady has an illness consisting of slow onset fever, myalgia, headache, cough, and constipation with leukopenia and mildly deranged LFT. She had a diarrhoeal illness in Pakistan, hinting at the possibility of another food- or water-borne illness. She has enteric fever.

The three most likely tropical infections are malaria, typhoid, and dengue.

- A malaria film is always the first investigation to think of in the returning traveller (cf *Book 3* –Haematology Questions 10, 11).
- Blood cultures are often positive for typhoid in the first week of illness (urine and stool thereafter) and will also pick up other illnesses presenting with bacteraemia. Lack of examination findings does not preclude use of a CXR.
- Dengue is a very common but usually self-limiting illness and serological tests can take many days to obtain.
- Hepatitis serology should be requested given her abnormal LFT but she has a very mild transaminitis only and the diagnosis is less likely. Acute atypical respiratory serology will be negative initially and a paired convalescent sample (in 4–6 weeks) is necessary to diagnose an infection.

2 **A** Oral ciprofloxacin

3 **E** Bone marrow aspiration and culture is a useful diagnostic test

Enteric fever (typhoid or paratyphoid fever) is a food – or water-borne illness found worldwide, especially in developing countries; it is usually caused by the Gram negative bacilli *Salmonella typhi* or

Salmonella paratyphi types A, B and C. Labelling enteric fever as a diarrhoeal illness is dangerous, diarrhoea is present in only 20–40% of cases and as such it can lead one a misdiagnosis; it is better to consider it as a potentially fatal septicaemic illness. The clinical features above (and in Chapter 2 case 43) are typical. The diarrhoea is often bloody and the rash is faint, pink, maculo-papular occurring on the trunk (rose spots, very hard to see unless the patient is white) in the second week, the abdomen can be tender, hepatosplenomegaly and a relative bradycardia may occur.

The fever progressive in stepwise fashion and is then sustained.

Complications arise from the second week onwards and include:

- Intestinal haemorrhage
- Perforation of the bowel
- Septic shock
- Renal failure with the nephritic syndrome
- Pneumonia
- Meningitis
- Septic arthritis
- Osteomyelitis
- Death occurs in 20% if untreated

Treatment

- Ciprofloxacin – first line in the UK, but resistance is developing
- Ampicillin
- Chloramphenicol – the traditional worldwide first line therapy
- Third generation cephalosporins or azithromycin are alternatives

Chronic carriage occurs in 1–2%, usually in the biliary tree or urinary tract and in this case treatment should be for at least 1 month. Cholecystectomy is an option to reduce chronic carriage in the biliary tree. Chronic carriage and enteric secretion are public health problems.

Prevention

- Safe eating and drinking habits while travelling – avoid raw, undercooked food, tap water and ice-cubes in drinks, do not eat fruit or vegetables that might have been washed in tap water unless you can peel them yourself.
- Vaccination – not 100% effective

Lifelong immunity after infection does not occur.

Case 11

1   D   *Leishmania braziliensis*

Leishmaniasis is found in about 90 countries. Transmission is by the bite of a sandfly (*Phlebotomus* in the Old World, *Lutzomyia* in the New World). The *Leishmania* species causing cutaneous leishmaniasis (CL) and the clinical picture vary between geographical areas.

Old world CL

- *Leishmania major, L. tropica, L. aethiopica* produce most cases, and also the *L. donovani* species complex, which also cause visceral leishmaniasis (VL).
- The commonest clinical picture is localised CL or 'oriental sore'. A blister appears after 2–4 weeks at the site of the bite. This enlarges and forms an ulcer with a raised border. The lesion resolves after some months leaving a scar. It may recur months later at the same site – 'chronic relapsing' or 'recidivans' CL.
- Occasionally a disseminated form, diffuse CL, occurs when the host has impaired immunity.

New world CL

- *Leishmania viannia* complex (eg *L.v. braziliensis, L.v. panamensis*), *L. mexicana*, and *L. amazonensis* cause several illnesses.
  'Chiclero ulcer' – a destructive lesion occurring on the ear or face caused by *L. mexicana*
  'Uta' – causes destructive scarring of children in Peru.
  L.v. braziliensis infection causes many small ulcers that spread along the lymphatics. This latter infection is important because years later it can evolve into mucocutanaeous CL in up to 5% of patients; it is also known as 'Espundia'. One sees progressive destruction of tissue beginning at the mucocutaneous junction of the nose; marked disfigurement and secondary bacterial infection occur.

Diagnosis is by microscopy and by culture of biopsy or smear of tissue fluid from lesion edge. The organism can be identified by PCR. Non-*viannia* infections resolve spontaneously. Treatment depends on patient preference because drugs are not without serious side-effects and inconvenience. *Leishmania viannia* infections need treatment to prevent mucocutaneous VL. The choice is between sodium stibogluconate and liposomal amophotericin B. (cf *Book 2* – Dermatology Question 11)

Case 12

1 **E** Dengue fever

This young businessman has a fever–arthralgia–rash syndrome after returning from India. The incubation period was 4–6 days.

- Yellow fever is excluded easily because it does not occur in Asia; it occurs in Africa and the Americas only.
- Malaria should always be part of the differential diagnosis whatever the symptoms and signs. However, the incubation period of *P. falciparum* is 7–14 days – longer in non-*falciparum* malaria, making it a less likely diagnosis in this case. Unless performed and interpreted by specialists, serological tests should not be relied on for malaria diagnosis. Antibody tests can remain positive for months or years after infection, hence a positive result only indicated previous infection in this case. Malaria should be excluded be three negative blood films.
- Acute hepatitis A and HIV infection are again excluded because of their incubation periods – 2–6 weeks and 2 weeks to 3 months, respectively.

Dengue virus is an arthropod-borne virus (arbovirus). Over 100 million cases of dengue fever occur per year throughout the tropics. It is spread by the day-biting *Aedes* mosquito, therefore bite avoidance is more difficult, cf malaria, which is transmitted by night-biting *Anopheles*.

- The incubation period is usually 2–8 days.
- One classically sees fever over 40°C, arthralgia, and a widespread maculo-papular rash. It is associated with retro-orbital headache and severe myalgia. Fever and other symptoms settle after a few days.
- Investigations reveal thrombocytopenia, neutrophilia and deranged LFT.
- Diagnosis is made by detection of IgM antibodies or by PCR.
- It is usually a self-limiting illness.
- Complications include hepatitic and encephalitic illnesses.
- Sequential infection by different serotypes (usually occurring in children in endemic areas) causes dengue haemorrhagic fever (DHF). When this occurs with DIC and circulatory failure it is termed dengue shock syndrome.
- No antiviral agent is available, therefore supportive treatment is all that is available for DHF. No vaccination is available.

Case 13

1 **A** She has a simple parapneumonic effusion

2 **D** Q fever

When assessing a pleural effusion.

- Protein and LDH – effusions can be classified as transudates if the protein is < 30 g/L and exudates if protein is >30 g/L if the serum protein is normal. If the serum protein is not 'normal' use Light's criteria. The pleural fluid is an exudate if one or more of the following criteria are met:
  Pleural fluid protein divided by serum protein >0.5
  Pleural fluid LDH divided by serum LDH >0.6
  Pleural fluid LDH more than two-thirds the upper limits of normal serum LDH.
- LDH – is a good marker of pleural inflammation. High concentrations (>1000 IU/L) occur with complicated parapneumonic effusions.
- Cell count – is normally <1/mm³. With a predominant lymphocytosis the most likely diagnoses are tuberculosis and malignancy. If polymorphonuclear cells predominate plus parenchymal shadowing, the most likely diagnoses are parapneumonic effusion or pulmonary embolism with infarction. If there is no parenchymal shadowing, the likely diagnoses are pulmonary embolism, viral infection, acute tuberculosis, or benign asbestos pleural effusion.
- pH – is normally c. 7.6. In an infected effusion a pH of <7.2 indicates need for tube drainage.
- Glucose – usually ≈ plasma glucose. Reduced levels indicate inflammation.

Causes of an exudative pleural effusion.

- Common causes
  Malignancy
  Parapneumonic effusions
- Less common causes
  Pulmonary infarction
  Rheumatoid arthritis
  Autoimmune diseases
  Benign asbestos effusion
  Pancreatitis
  Post-myocardial infarction syndrome
- Rare causes
  Yellow nail syndrome
  Drugs, eg amiodarone, nitrofurantoin, phenytoin
  Fungal infections.

Causes of a transudative pleural effusion.

- Very common causes

       Left ventricular failure
       Liver cirrhosis
       Hypoalbuminaemia
       Peritoneal dialysis
- Less common causes
       Hypothyroidism
       Nephrotic syndrome
       Mitral stenosis
       Pulmonary embolism
- Rare causes
       Constrictive pericarditis
       Urinothorax
       Superior vena cava obstruction
       Ovarian hyperstimulation
       Meigs syndrome.

Following pneumonia, an empyema may form beginning with a simple exudative effusion. This simple parapneumonic effusion, as in this patient, has a pH >7.20, LDH <1000 U/L, glucose >2.2 mmol/L, and no organisms on Gram stain. It can be managed with appropriate antibiotics. A complicated parapneumonic effusion, the next stage, would be suggested by pH <7.20, LDH > 1000 U/L, glucose >2.2 mmol/L, with/without organisms on Gram stain and requires chest tube drainage. As does an empyema in which frank pus is aspirated with organisms on Gram stain.[3,4]

This patient has recently visited a farm or petting zoo. The most likely cause is Q fever caused by *Coxiella burnetii*, a zoonosis spread by aerosol or direct contact. Sheep, cows, and goats are the usual reservoir. It can present as an atypical pneumonia and occasionally it is complicated by effusion. Other presentations include hepatitis (in 50%), pleuropericarditis, myocarditis and meningoencephalitis.

Pneumonia can occur in brucellosis and leptospirosis but these differentials are less likely. *Nocardia* causes a cavitating pneumonia with empyema, but is almost exclusive to immunosupressed patients or those with chronic chest disease.

Case 14

1   **B**   Daily operations will be required
     D   Hyperbaric oxygen therapy may be of benefit

This injecting drug user has necrotising fasciitis. He is septic and hypotensive and requires urgent management.

Necrotising fasciitis is a rare but devastating illness. There are two forms.

- Type 1 is caused by a mixed anaerobic and aerobic infection. It usually complicates operations or occurs in diabetic patients or those with peripheral vascular disease.
- Type 2 is caused by group A streptococci and occurs in the previously fit and well, sometimes spontaneously or after an innocuous blunt injury or muscle strain. It also occurs in injecting drug users and following penetrating injuries.

Clinically it may be difficult to pick up. Infections begin in the deep tissues and spread along fascial planes and early signs may be minimal with clinical features of cellulitis. However, pain is often severe and out of proportion to external signs. There is rapid progression. The skin darkens and develops bullae. When this occurs there is already massive destruction of deeper tissues. The patient is toxic and unwell.

Laboratory findings will include a neutrophilia and elevated CK. MRI can differentiate between cellulitis and necrotising fasciitis in difficult cases.

Urgent surgical debridement is required. It may not be possible to stabilise the patient before theatre and delay in operating will result in an increased mortality. Repeated operations will be required (a mean of four in injecting drug users with necrotising fasciitis). Clindamycin suppresses toxin production by the organisms and has some anaerobic cover; it is usually given with penicillin; iv immunoglobulin can be administered as it may contain neutralising antibodies. Hyperbaric therapy has been used in this infection, usually when involving the head and neck and multiple case reports show a benefit.

Drotrecogin-alpha is discussed elsewhere (see Case 16, this section).

Case 15

1 **D** Bot fly larva

The bot fly is a resident of South America. The fly lays eggs on a smaller blood sucking fly. When this fly is feeding on human blood the heat causes the egg to hatch; the larva falls onto the skin and then burrows under the skin. Here, the larva grows within the host but does not invade beyond the subcutaneous tissues. It is itchy or painful, particularly as the larva enlarges and moves, the bot fly larva has spines. Forty to fifty days later it eventually emerges as an adult fly. Many are inadvertently removed, such as in this case. Others where identified can be smothered with petroleum jelly or a non-porous dressing. The maggot's spiracles, its breathing apparatus, are blocked and the larva tries to emerge. It can then be eased out with forceps. An alternative to this – in some parts of the world – is to apply fatty bacon over the wound and secure with a dressing, the bot fly prefers the bacon to the human flesh and migrates into it, whereupon it can be grasped with tweezers and fully removed!

- *Ancylostoma braziliense* is a dog hookworm whose larvae cause cutaneous larva migrans.
- *Chrysomyia* fly larvae, 'screw worms', cause invasive myiasis – an invasive maggot disease. Maggots destroy healthy skin and soft tissue and can invade into deep structures, eg the nasal sinuses or, rather disturbingly, the brain.
- The Tumbu fly lives in Africa. It lays its eggs on drying clothes. When worn, the eggs hatch and the maggots penetrate the skin, causing small lesions similar to those of the bot fly. Ironing clothes before wearing destroys the eggs.
- *Tunga penetrans* is a flea. These 'chiggers' penetrate the skin, usually the foot, causing local itching and bacterial superinfection.
- The Guinea worm is an invasive tissue nematode worm causing dracunculiasis. The female adult worms may reach lengths of >100 cm before emerging through the skin of the legs. It occurs in Africa only.

Case 16

1   A   *Staphylococcus aureus*

2   C   Consideration of drotecogin – alpha therapy

This lady has staphylococcal toxic shock syndrome (TSS). A similar illness can be caused by toxin-producing group A streptococci. While the other organisms in the question can cause a septicaemic illness with multiple organ involvement, she fulfils the criteria described below and has had an IUCD inserted recently. Cases of TSS have been reported in this setting and can complicate any focal staphylococcal infection, although most are in association with menstruation and the use of tampons. The illness is the result of a massive inflammatory response triggered by toxins. Toxic shock syndrome toxin 1 (TSST-1) is associated with 90% of menstrual cases and 50% of non-menstrual cases; staphylococcal enterotoxin B (SEB) is found in the remainder of TSST-1-negative cases.

TSS is often a clinical diagnosis. Blood cultures are positive in only 5–10% of cases and other causes need to be excluded. Treatment involves supportive therapy and antibiotics, eg iv flucloxacillin and clindamycin for 1 week. Antibiotics do not alter the clinical course, but do prevent recurrence. Remove the source of toxin if possible.

Criteria for diagnosis of toxic shock (from Centre of Disease Control)

Patients require all of the following:

- Fever – >38.9°C
- Rash – diffuse macular erythroderma which should desquamate after 1–2 weeks
- Hypotension – systolic blood pressure ≤90 mmHg
- Multisystem involvement – need three or more of:
  Gastrointestinal – vomiting or diarrhoea at onset of illness
  Muscular – severe myalgia or creatine phosphokinase ≥2× normal
  Renal – urea or creatinine ≥ 2× normal, or pyuria in absence of UTI
  Hepatic – abnormal LFT
  Platelets – ≤100,000/mL
  CNS – disoriented or alterations in consciousness without focal neurological signs when fever and hypotension are absent.

Activated protein C (APC) is an endogenous protein that modulates and inhibits thrombosis and inflammation in severe sepsis. Sepsis reduces the level of protein C and inhibits conversion of protein C to APC. Drotrecogin-alpha (recombinant APC) when used in severe sepsis resulted in lower mortality rates (PROWESS study[5]). It should be considered for patients presenting with severe sepsis. The main side-effect is increased risk of bleeding.

In suspected cases of meningococcal septicaemia, even if meningism is present, a lumbar puncture should not be performed because of the risk of haemorrhage and because it adds little to the diagnosis and management.

Case 17

1   **D**   Visceral leishmaniasis

Visceral leishmaniasis (VL) is usually caused by species from the *Leishmania donovani* complex (*L. donovani*, *L. chagasi*, and *L. infantum*). Occasionally, the *L. braziliensis* complex is involved. While VL occurs across the world, with 90% of cases occurring in the Indian subcontinent, Afghanistan, Brazil, and Sudan, it is also endemic to southern Europe. Most cases here are transmitted by sandflies (likely in this case) but blood-borne transmission between intravenous drug users is common, with many infections occurring in HIV-infected patients.

Following an incubation period of 2–12 months, the patient develops an insidious illness of fever, weight loss, night sweats, and abdominal discomfort. Lymphadenopathy, hepatomegaly, and moderate/massive splenomegaly are found on examination. Laboratory findings include anaemia as a result of bone marrow infiltration and splenic sequestration. Thrombocytopenia and leukopenia, hypoalbuminaemia, and polyclonal hypergammaglobulinaemia are common.

Diagnosis is made by demonstration of amastigotes (Leishman–Donovan bodies) on biopsy or culture specimens.

- Bone marrow biopsy has the highest yield (qv *Book 3* – Haematology Question 8).
- Liver and lymph nodes investigations are also useful.
- Culture should use NNN media.
- Serological tests are highly sensitive and specific, eg K39 ELISA, IFAT.
- Speciation can be performed by PCR of tissue or a culture specimen.

Without treatment, VL has a mortality >90%.

- The standard drug of choice is iv sodium stibogluconate (a pentavalent antimonial).
- An alternative is liposomal amphotericin B.
- Miltefosine, an oral agent, may be used in the future.

Case 18

1   C   Diphtheria

2   D   iv diphtheria anti-toxin

This young man has pharyngitis with extensive exudates, conduction abnormality on his ECG (second-degree heart block). He possibly has a 'bull neck' and palatal paralysis.

Infection by *Corynebacterium diphtheriae* is rare in the UK because of childhood vaccination. Most UK cases are the result of imported infections – recent major outbreaks have occurred in Eastern Europe and ex-USSR states.

Spread is via respiratory droplets or contact with infected saliva. The organisms usually remain in the respiratory mucosa. Cutaneous diphtheria ('veld sore' or 'desert sore') is sometimes seen. The clinical syndrome, once called the 'strangling angel of children' is largely the result of a potent exotoxin that inhibits protein synthesis and causes local tissue necrosis. The incubation period is 2–5 days.

Local features

- A necrotic mass of tissue, organisms, and inflammatory cells forms an extensive and adherent grey/green/black 'pseudomembrane'. This pseudomembrane and toxin-induced palatal paralysis can cause respiratory obstruction. Local oedema and lymphadenopathy cause a 'bull neck' appearance.

Systemic features

- The toxin is absorbed and causes cardiotoxicity (50–70% deaths), with conduction disturbances (complete AV dissociation and VT can occur) and heart failure, demyelination of nerves (cranial nerve palsies, dysphagia, paralysis, coma), and renal toxicity. Neurological signs often develop late, from 10 days to 3 months.

The diagnosis is made by culture from pharyngeal and nasal swabs. A toxin test can be performed (Elek test) and PCR is available.

Treatment

- iv diphtheria anti-toxin (equine) must be administered as soon as possible. Delay results in a poorer prognosis.
- The patient needs cardiac monitoring; early intubation and ventilation should be considered.
- iv penicillin or erythromycin should be administered for 14 days; they halt toxin production and eradicate organisms; they are not a substitute for anti-toxin.

Differential diagnoses:

- This patient does not fulfil the criteria for diagnosis of rheumatic fever (cf Book 1 – Cardiology Question 23).
- Miller–Fisher syndrome is an uncommon variant of Guillain-Barré syndrome – up to 5% of cases – and causes ophthalmoplegia and ataxia. Dysphagia and cardiac arrythmias can occur; the onset is usually post-infectious.
- CCHF is a viral haemorrhagic fever spread by ticks. Epidemics occur in the Balkans, Russia, the Middle East and Africa. One sees fever, neck pain, meningoencephalitis, then haemorrhagic phenomena. The condition is fatal in up to 30%. Ribavarin reduces mortality.
- Fusobacterium necrophorum is a Gram-negative anaerobic bacillus that causes a severe sore throat with septicaemia; it is known as Lemierre syndrome or necrobacillosis. There is often pleuropulmonary dissemination. Cardiac manifestations are not seen.

The UK childhood immunisation schedule is outlined below[6]:

Age	Vaccinations	No. injections
2, 3 and 4 months old	Diphtheria, tetanus, pertussis, polio and Hib (DTaP/IPV/Hib)	1
	Meningitis C	1
Around 13 months old	Measles, mumps and rubella (MMR)	1
3 years to 5 years old	Diphtheria, tetanus, pertussis, polio (dTaP/IPV or DTaP/IPV)	1
	Measles, mumps and rubella (MMR)	1
13–18 years old	Diphtheria, tetanus, polio (Td/IPV)	1

Note. The current universal BCG vaccination programme is to be replaced with a programme of targeted vaccination for those individuals who are at greatest risk.

Case 19

1   C   *Bartonella henselae*

Bartonella henselae causes cat scratch disease, a common cause of regional lymphadenopathy in young people. Ninety per cent of patients recall contact with cats, especially kittens, though not all will recall the injury. After an incubation of 3–10 days a papular rash develops close to the site of inoculation. Localised adenopathy then occurs. The skin is often red, and the node(s) can suppurate, causing sinuses. Generalised lymphadenopathy can occur. Occasional spread occurs to the reticulo-endothelial system and distant organs, eg CNS, lungs (<1%).

Diagnosis is made by biopsy. Granuloma and microabscess formation with Gram-negative rods (Warthin–Starry stain) is seen. Serology and PCR are also available as diagnostic techniques.

It is a self-limiting illness in the immunocompetent. The nodes resolve after 4–6 weeks, but may persist for 1 year. Treatment is reserved for persistent or generalised disease, and the immunocompromised. Various combinations of rifampicin, doxycycline, co-trimoxazole, ciprofloxacin, and gentamicin are used.

- *Francisella tularensis* and *Bacillus anthracis* have been mentioned frequently in the media over recent years as possible agents of bioterrorism.
- Ulceroglandular and glandular tularaemia are the commonest patterns of infection with *Francisella tularensis*. Usually they occur via percutaneous spread from animals (rabbits, hares). Patients are ill with severe constitutional symptoms and infiltrates visible on CXR. There is also inhalational and food-borne spread. The mortality is up to 30%. Treatment is with either streptomycin or gentamycin.
- *Chlamydia trachomatis* (serovars L1, L2, L3) causes lymphogranuloma venereum.
- *Capnocytophaga canimorsus* infection causes wound infection after animal bites. Severe sepsis is seen in post-splenectomy patients and alcoholics. Treatment is with co-amoxiclav or co-trimoxazole and metronidazole.

Normal lymph nodes are not palpable, except for inguinal nodes.

Infectious causes of lymphadenopathy

- Generalised bacterial
  B. henselae – cat scratch disease
  Brucella spp. – brucellosis
  Francisella tularensis – tularaemia
  Mycobacterium tuberculosis
  Mycobacterium avium intercellulare

- Localised bacterial
    Bacterial lymphadenitis
    B. anthracis –anthrax
    Y. pestis – plague
    Mycobacterium tuberculosis
    Mycobacterium leprae
    Chlamydia trachomatis – lymphogranuloma venereum
    B. henselae – cat scratch disease
- Fungal
    Histoplasma
    Coccidioides
    Paracoccidioides
- Viral
    EBV
    CMV
    HIV
- Parasitic
    Toxoplasma gondii
    Filiariasis

Non-infectious causes of lymphadenopathy

- Inflammatory
    Systemic lupus erythematosus
    Rheumatoid arthritis
    Sarcoidosis
    Amyloidosis
- Malignancy
    Metastatic – lung, breast, stomach, thyroid cancers
- Haematological malignancy
    Lymphoma
    Leukaemia
    Multiple myeloma
    (Castleman's disease)
- Drugs – phenytoin
- Inherited – Gaucher's disease.

Case 20

1   **C**   Leptospirosis

See answer to Chapter 2, Case 41 pages 155 and 156.

Case 21

1   **A**   Blood cultures
    B   Transthoracic echocardiogram (TTE)
    D   Stereotactic brain biopsy

2   **D**   Cerebral abscess

A young woman with clubbing, cyanosis, and a heart murmur presents with a generalised seizure and a mass on CT scan. She is febrile with a neutrophilia. The most likely diagnosis is a cerebral abscess. She has congenital heart disease with a right-to-left shunt (Eisenmenger syndrome).

Brain abscesses occur following:

- Direct invasion from a contiguous source, eg sinusitis, otitis media
- Recent trauma or neurosurgery
- Metastatic spread from a distant focus, eg endocarditis, lung abscess
- A common association in children is congenital heart disease, especially if right-to-left shunt is present.

The cause is mixed organisms in 50% of cases: they include *Staphylococcus aureus, Streptococcus milleri, Streptococcus pneumoniae*, coliforms, *Haemophilus influenzae*, anaerobic Gram-positive cocci, *Actinomyces* spp.

Diagnosis

- Patients present with a subacute history (often 1–4 weeks) of increasing headache and signs of an intracranial mass, eg localising signs, signs of raised intracranial pressure, seizures. Only around 50% have fever.
- Imaging with CT or MRI scan shows ring-enhancing lesion(s) with oedema.
- A lumbar pucture is **always** contraindicated because of the risk of herniation of the brainstem (coning).
- Blood cultures should be taken, as should specimens from sites of distant infection.
- A peripheral neutrophilia is usual.

Treatment

- When an abscess has been demonstrated the neurosurgeons should be asked to aspirate it either with stereotactic guidance or at craniotomy.
- Aspiration is important diagnostically and for treatment – only small abscesses should be treated with antibiotics alone.

The initial antibiotic choice is iv cefotaxime 2–4 g 8-hourly plus iv metronidazole 500 mg 8-hourly. Thereafter modify regimen when specific bacteriology is available (cf *Chapter 2, Case 47 page 161* and *Book 1* – Cardiology Questions 20, 30, 31).

A TTE is useful given the patient's underlying condition and to exclude endocarditis. The patient's lymphocyte count is 1.5×10^9/L suggesting a normal CD4 count. HIV infection with opportunistic infection or tumour is unlikely. A tuberculoma is an unlikely diagnosis given the lack of epidemiological clues in the question.

A CXR should be performed but will not add to the diagnosis.

Case 22

1   **E**   Tetanus

2   **B**   Nursing in a quiet environment
    C   Human anti-tetanus immunoglobulin

Tetanus is caused by the Gram-positive anaerobe *Clostridium tetani*, a spore-forming organism found in soil, dust, and faeces. It can remain in tissue for months. A rare disease in the UK because of immunisation, it is occasionally seen in the elderly who are often unvaccinated. Clostridial infections, including *C. tetani*, *C. botulinum*, and *C. novyi* (which caused a severe septic illness with high case fatality rate in 2000) have caused outbreaks in injecting drug users over the past few years. Always think about these infections in an injecting drug user with lesions from 'skin popping' ie injection into subcutaneous tissue or muscle (as shown in the picture).

Patients with generalised tetanus present with trismus (masseter spasm), restlessness, fever, dysphagia, and back pain because of muscle spasm. Violent, painful, muscle spasms become increasingly frequent and generalised and can be triggered by noise or touch; these can cause fractures and can eventually lead to respiratory failure.

The diagnosis is clinical although the organism can be cultured from wounds. Patients should be managed on ITU where they can be intubated and ventilated if required, and high doses of benzodiazepines and neuromuscular blockade (eg infusion of pancuronium) can be given. One must beware of sympathetic overactivity – the major cause of death on ITU, which is treated with labetolol.

Treatment of tetanus is with anti-tetanus immunoglobulin im at multiple sites, iv metronidazole or benzylpenicillin, and wound debridement; tetanus vaccination should be commenced.

The mortality is up to 5–50% despite ITU.

- The only differential diagnosis for tetanus is strychnine poisoning.
- Dental infections, tumours, and hysteria can all mimic trismus.
- There is no indication for a lumbar puncture.
- Botulism causes an illness characterised by a symmetrical, descending paralysis with autonomic disturbance in an afebrile patient.

- Guillain–Barré syndrome causes a flaccid, ascending paralysis.
- Tetanus does not cause paralysis.
- There are no clinical findings or evidence of cardiotoxicity to suggest diphtheria. (cf *Book 3* – Neurology Question 1).

Case 23

1 **A** Yellow fever virus
   B *Wuchereria bancrofti*
   D Dengue virus
   J Japanese encephalitis virus
   K *Brugia malayi*
   P West Nile virus
   Q *Plasmodium malariae*

The picture shows a mosquito (actually an *Aedes* mosquito but the features distinguishing it from an *Anopheles* mosquito are not relevant here). Knowledge of simple vector biology is helpful in making a differential diagnosis of fever in the returning traveller.

Vector	Infection	Organism
Mosquito	Malaria	*Plasmodium falciparum* *Plasmodium vivax* *Plasmodium ovale* *Plasmodium malariae*
	Filiariasis	*Wuchereria bancrofti* *Brugia malayi/ timori*
	Arboviruses	Dengue virus Yellow fever virus West Nile virus Japanese B encephalitis
Blackfly (*Simulium*)	Onchocerciasis	*Onchocerca volvulus*
Deerfly (*Chrysops*)	Loa loiasis	*Loa loa*
Sandfly (*Phlebotomus, Lutzomyia*)	Leishmaniasis Sandfly fever	*Leishmania* spp. Phlebovirus
Tsetse fly	African trypanosomiasis ('Sleeping sickness')	*Trypanosoma brucei*
Tick	Lyme disease Endemic relapsing fever Tularaemia Ehrlichiosis Rocky mountain spotted fever Arboviruses	*Borrelia burgdorferi* *Borrelia* spp. *Francisella tularensis* *Ehrlichia chaffeensis* *Rickettsia rickettsii* Congo-Crimean HF virus Colorado tick fever

Table (*continued*)

Vector	Infection	Organism
	Babesiosis	*Babesia* spp
Reduviid bug	American trypanosomiasis (Chagas' disease)	*Trypanosoma cruzi*
Flea	Plague	*Yersinia pestis*
	Endemic/murine typhus	*Rickettsia typhi*
Louse	Epidemic relapsing fever	*Borrelia recurrentis*
	Epidemic typhus	*Rickettsia prowazekii*
	Trench fever	*Bartonella quintana*
Mites	Scrub typhus	*Rickettsia tsutsugamushi*

Lassa fever virus is spread by contact with urine from the multimammate mouse. Contact with rodent excreta also transmits hantaviruses (which cause a severe pulmonary-renal syndrome). The route of Ebola (and Marburg) virus transmission is unknown.

Case 24

1   **B**   Acute viral myocarditis

A young patient presents with congestive heart failure following a flu-like illness. Her ECG shows ST elevation in both the inferior and anterior leads. She most likely has a viral myocarditis.

Myocarditis is inflammation of the myocardium with myocyte necrosis. It usually manifests in the young and fit. It has many causes including:

- Toxins – drug hypersensitivity, cocaine, toxins, radiation
- Autoimmune – systemic lupus erythematosus, rheumatoid arthritis, vasculitis
- Inflammatory – sarcoid, rheumatic fever
- Peripartum
- Up to 50% of cases are idiopathic

Infectious causes include:

- Viral
    Enteroviruses (coxsackie B, coxsackie A, echovirus)
    Influenza virus A and B
    Rubella virus, mumps virus
    CMV, EBV
    Adenovirus
- Bacterial
    Coxiella burnetii
    Leptospira spp.

> *Borrelia* spp. (Lyme disease)
> *Mycoplasma pneumoniae*
> Syphilis
> • Parasite
> Trypanosomiasis – Chagas' disease
> *Toxoplasma gondii*
> Malaria.

In viral myocarditis there is usually a history of a 'viral illness' in the preceding 2 weeks. Symptoms include increasing fatigue, dyspnoea, palpitations, and chest pain. Examination findings include fever, tachycardia, arrhythmias, or features of heart failure. ECG changes are variable but may show ST elevation or inversion, and T-wave changes in all leads. Ventricular ectopics, dysrhythmias and AV block may be seen. Laboratory studies reveal elevated CK and Troponin I or T. Enterovirus can occasionally be cultured from throat or stool specimens. Otherwise the diagnosis is made with serological tests (detection of an antibody rise in convalescent blood samples). No specific treatment is available and often it resolves completely. However, it may rarely be severe enough to result in a cardiomyopathy warranting heart transplant.

Myocarditis occurs in early disseminated Lyme disease, weeks or months after the tick bite. Although the patient does not mention if she was walking in South America, myocarditis in Chagas' disease occurs years after infection with *Trypanosoma cruzi*. Although the illness has occurred after an upper respiratory illness there, the case does not meet the Modified Jones criteria for rheumatic fever (cf *Book 1* – Cardiology Question 23). This needs two major or one major and two minor criteria to diagnose rheumatic fever.

Major criteria	Minor criteria
Carditis – pancarditis	Fever
Arthritis – large joint, migratory	Arthralgia
Chorea – 'St Vitus's dance', erratic, purposeless movements	Raised CRP or ESR
Subcutaneous nodules – crops over bony prominences	Previous RF
Erythema marginatum – pink, serpiginous, non-tender	Prolonged PR interval

Case 25

1   **D**   iv tazocin – (piperacillin and tazobactam)

2   **E**   Graft-versus-host disease (GVHD) is unlikely

3   **A**   An iv glycopeptide should be added to the regimen

This gentleman is profoundly neutropenic following an allogeneic bone marrow transplant (BMT) and has developed a febrile illness (cf. *Book 3* – Haematology Question 5). He has a mucositis making him prone to invasion from microbes and his Hickman line is inflamed.

A 'febrile neutropenic episode' can be defined as an oral temperature of $>38°C$ for >1 h in association with a neutrophil count $<1.0 \times 10^9/L$. Most cases will be seen in patients with haematological malignancy receiving chemotherapy, and most will be the result of infection. Non-infectious causes need to be excluded:

- Underlying pathology – neoplasm, tumour necrosis
- Drugs – cyclophosphamide, cytarabine, hydroxyurea
- Antimicrobials – amphotericin
- Transfusion of blood products
- Inflammation – thromboembolic disease, thrombophlebitis, haematoma.

BMT involves the harvesting of haematopoietic stem cells from a donor's blood or bone marrow.

- Allogeneic transplant – from another person
- Syngeneic transplant – an identical twin
- Autologous transplant – from the patient themselves

These stem cells are infused into the recipient who has had chemotherapy (with or without irradiation), which depletes the recipient's bone marrow. This can result in profound neutropenia.

The risk of bacterial and fungal sepsis increases exponentially when the neutrophil count is $<0.5 \times 10^9/L$. Infective agents are usually Gram-positive bacteria (although historically enterobacteriaceae and *Pseudomonas aeruginosa*) and fungi – *Aspergillus* spp. by inhalation or *Candida* spp. by invasion.

Preventative measures include

- Prophylactic antibiotics – the recommendations vary. Fluoroquinolones reduce infection-related mortality, therefore they are used in patients with anticipated prolonged or severe neutropenia. Fungal prophylaxis is usually aimed at *Candida* spp., that cross damaged mucosal surfaces, amphotericin, fluconazole, voriconazole are all used.
- Protective isolation – use of single rooms with positive pressure ventilation and HEPA filtration and barrier-nursing methods.

Patients with neutropenic sepsis may present with a paucity of symptoms and signs. Sources of infection are identified in $>80–90\%$ by microbiological sampling from sputum, wounds, indwelling vascular and urinary catheters, and peripheral blood cultures.

Treatment

- This is initially empirical, with broad-spectrum antimicrobials that cover pseudomonads. This has resulted in a decreased mortality in neutropenic patients, especially following BMT.
- Use extended spectrum penicillin with β-lactamase inhibitor, eg tazocin (piperacillin and tazobactam), timentin (ticarcillin and clavulanate), fluoroquinolone, third- and fourth-generation cephalosporins (ceftazidime, cefixime) either as monotherapy or in combination with an aminoglycoside (gentamycin, amikacin).
- Fever may take a median of 5 days to resolve, despite the correct antibiotics. However, a patient with a fever after 3–4 days should be still be reassessed with further clinical sampling and imaging. Granulocyte transfusion should be considered in culture-positive Gram-negative sepsis not responsive to antibiotics if the neutropaenia continues.
- Empirical antifungal therapy, eg liposomal amphotericin B, should be commenced if there is no identifiable source of infection and if the neutrophil count is not expected to recover in the next 5–7 days.
- In a proven Gram-positive infection, antibiotics are continued for 10–14 days, at least 14 days in a Gram-negative infection and for 5 days after fever resolves in culture-negative cases. In some units antibiotics are continued until 4–5 days after neutrophil counts recover.

In our case a glycopeptide should be added (vancomycin, teicoplanin) to cover coagulase-negative staphylococcus, MRSA, and enterococci that may be causing a line site infection. Intravascular lines are usually removed when there are proven mycobacterial and fungal infections of the device. Gram-negative infections (*Pseudomonas*, *Acinetobacter*) often warrant removal because of a low likelihood of successful treatment. Our patient has no evidence of these. CMV infection and GVHD are complications that usually occur ≥1 month following BMT.

Case 26

1   **D**   Epstein–Barr virus infection

2   **C**   He should avoid contact sports for at least 1 month.

This young man has an illness characteristic of infectious mononucleosis (IM). The commonest cause (90% of cases) is Epstein–Barr virus (EBV). Non-EBV causes include cytomegalovirus (CMV), herpes simplex viruses 1 and 2 (HSV-1 and -2), human herpesvirus 6 (HHV-6), hepatitis A, B, and C viruses, *Toxoplasma gondii*, adenovirus, rubella, and acute HIV infection.

EBV is very common. Most cases occur in young children (>50% in <5-year-olds) and go unnoticed. Young adults (15–24 years) not exposed to EBV previously can develop IM. Spread is via saliva and respiratory secretions. Only 5–10% is the result of contact with a known IM patient. After 30–50 days incubation the patient develops fever, sore throat, lymphadenopathy, headache and abdominal discomfort. Sore throat is maximal for the first 5 days. Symptoms resolve after 2–3 weeks. The signs include splenomegaly in 50%, hepatomegaly in 20%, and rash in 10%. Complications include anaemia and thrombocytopenia, splenic rupture (spontaneous 50%, traumatic 50%), meningoencephalitis, and Guillain–Barré syndrome. EBV-associated malignancies include Burkitt's lymphoma, nasopharyngeal carcinoma, and lymphoproliferative disease in immunosuppressed patients (B-cell lymphoma in HIV infection, post-transplant lymphoproliferative disease).

Laboratory abnormalities include a transaminitis and a lymphocytosis (of 10×10^9 to 25×10^9/L) with aytipical lymphocytes on the blood film. The causes of atypical lymphocytosis are the same as the causes of IM.

Diagnosis is by detection of heterophile antibodies (polyclonal antibodies that agglutinate cells from animals), eg Paul–Bunnell and Monospot tests, or EBV serology (including EBNA and VCA antibodies). Infection results in lifelong immunity.

Very rarely infection can persist as a chronic active infection. (This is not to be confused with post-viral chronic fatigue syndrome.) The outlook of chronic active infection is poor with few patients living more than 10 years after diagnosis – the main mortality is from lymphoproliferative disorders and bone marrow failure.

Case 27

1   E   Acute pulmonary histoplasmosis

See answer to Chapter 2, Case 48 pages 161 and 162.

Sarcoidosis is less likely given the rapid onset and the patient being male.

Legionella pneumonia is unlikely because, if the illness is connected to his holiday, the incubation period is too long; incubation period is 2–10 days for *L. pneumophilia* (qv Ch 1 question 20).

The patient seems well despite extensive CXR changes which is often seen in histoplasmosis

The patient is married, and (unless he was 'a businessman on a foreign trip'!) should not have HIV in the MRCP examination, furthermore the onset is too rapid.

There are again no epidemiological clues suggesting miliary tuberculosis and the onset is rapid (qv Book 2 Gastroenterology question 10).

Case 28

1   B   *Burkholderia pseudomallei*

This lady has melioidosis as a result of *Burkholderia pseudomallei* infection. She has presented weeks later with a cavitating pneumonia and profound weight loss after visiting South-east Asia.

The Gram-negative bacillus *B. pseudomallei* is a soil saprophyte often found in rice paddy fields. It is a common cause of septicaemia in South-east Asia and is also found in northern Australia. Spread is by inoculation or inhalation. Patients can present months, or even years, after exposure with septicaemia or localised infection, usually in the lung; occasionally abscesses occur in bone, liver, spleen, parotid glands or the prostate after septicaemic spread. The infection is often subclinical and relapse is recognised.

Diagnosis is made by microscopy of specimens and culture on selective media. Serology by CFT is the most specific test and PCR is available.

The treatment is prolonged, initially with high-dose oral or iv co-trimoxazole plus iv ceftazidime (or a carbapenem) for 14 days. Treatment may, however, be up to 8 weeks in deep-seated infections, followed by 3–6 months of oral co-trimoxazole (high dose) or augmentin (amoxicillin and clavulanate).

- *Mycobacterium tuberculosis* may cause a similar illness but mycobacteria are Gram-positive rods.
- The fungus *Penicillium marneffei* causes a progressive and disseminated infection (penicilliosis) in immunocompromised patients in China and South-east Asia.
- *Cryptococcus neoformans* can cause a cavitating pneumonia in the immunocompromised.
- *Pseudomonas aeruginosa* is of the same genus as *B. pseudomallei* but causes pneumonia in immunocompromised, ventilated or neutropenic patients, and those with chronic chest disease. There is nothing to suggest infection in the history.

	Gram positive Aerobes	Anaerobes	Gram-negative Aerobes	Anaerobes
Cocci	Staphylococci Streptococci		Neisseria Moraxella	
Rods	Bacillus Listeria Mycobacterium Nocardia Corynebacterium	Clostridium Actinomyces	Enterobacteriaceae Escherichia Proteus Klebsiella Enterobacter Pseudomonas Haemophilus Salmonella Shigella Brucella Bordetella	Bacteroides Fusobacterium
Curved rods			Vibrio Campylobacter Helicobacter (microaerophiles)	
Spirochaetes*	Treponema Leptospira Borrelia			

* Stain poorly with Gram's stain

Case 29

1   E   Squamous cell carcinoma of lung

The patient is a chronic smoker with clubbing, hyponatraemia, and a cavitating lesion in his right lung (cf *Book 1* – Respiratory Question 23). The history may suggest a diagnosis of TB or an aspergilloma within an old TB cavity but the likely diagnosis is bronchial carcinoma.

Aspergillus species are moulds found in organic matter. The main human pathogenic species are *Aspergillus fumigatus, A. niger, A. flavus* and *A. clavatus*; transmission is via inhalation.

There are four main pulmonary syndromes:

- ABPA
- Chronic necrotising *Aspergillus* pneumonia, in steroid-dependent COPD and alcoholics
- Invasive aspergillosis in patients with immunodeficiency and prolonged neutropenia

- Aspergilloma – in the severely immunocompromised *Aspergillus* may spread haematogenously to kidney, liver, heart, eye, spleen, soft tissue, and bone.

An aspergilloma is a mycetoma (fungal ball); it develops in a pre-existing cavity within lung parenchyma, usually an old TB scar. It may move within the cavity but does not invade the cavity wall. Haemoptysis occurs in 40–60%, which can be massive and life-threatening. They may cause cough and fever.

The diagnosis of aspergillosis usually requires microbiological or histopathological evidence of an organism. Radiological imaging can be characteristic in an aspergilloma. *Aspergillus* precipitin antibody test results are usually positive. Galactomannan is a polysaccharide released from *Aspergillus* during growth, detected using EIA or PCR tests; it is of use in the diagnosis of invasive aspergillosis and may be positive in aspergilloma.

The treatment is by surgical resection if the patient is symptomatic. Anti-fungals are used if surgery is not an option. Oral itraconazole may provide partial or complete resolution of aspergillomas in 60% of patients. Intracavitary amphotericin and acetylcysteine or aminocaproic acid have been used with some success.

Case 30

1   **E**   Doxycycline 100 mg daily

2   **B**   Diphtheria and tetanus toxoid
     D   Injectable typhoid
     E   Hepatitis A

This lady is immunosuppressed (rheumatoid arthritis, prednisolone, and methotrexate) but is planning travel to a tropical country. She is taking antidepressants.

Repeated malaria infections during childhood will have conferred partial immunity to the patient so reducing the severity of illness, but as she has lived in a non-endemic area for many years her immunity will have waned. The recommendation would be to take chemoprophylaxis and to avoid bites (mosquito net, insect repellent containing a high concentration of DEET, wearing long sleeves and trousers after dusk). Malarone (atovaquone/ proguanil) and doxycycline would be the two recommended choices. Mefloquine is very useful but is contraindicated because of her psychiatric history (depression). Resistance to chloroquine is widespread in Africa.

All travellers should have their diphtheria, polio, and tetanus vaccination status reviewed regardless of destination. Details of the recommended vaccinations for specific countries are beyond the scope of the MRCP examination (immunisation guidelines can be found in ref. 7). However, in general, patients should also be offered hepatitis A and typhoid vaccinations if travelling to countries where there is concern regarding hygiene and sanitation.

Below is a list of vaccinations available to travellers.

Live vaccines	Inactivated vaccines
MMR	Diphtheria toxoid
Oral poliomyelitis	Tetanus toxoid
Oral typhoid	Pertussis
BCG (TB)	*Haemophilus influenzae* b (Hib)
	Influenza
	Pneumococcal
	Hepatitis A
	Hepatitis B
	Typhoid (Injectable)
	Meningococcal (A&C)
	Japanese encephalitis
	Tick-borne encephalitis
	Rabies

Live vaccines are contraindicated in immunosuppressed patients. Therefore, yellow fever and oral polio vaccines should not be given to this patient (cf answer to Chapter 1, Case 9 pages 101 and 102). Hepatitis B would not be routinely offered unless a person was likely to be exposed to blood and bodily fluids, eg if planning to work in health care.

Case 31

1   **C**   African tick-bite fever (*Rickettsia africae*)

This lesion with central necrosis is an eschar or 'tache noire'. An eschar forms after a bite from a tick infected with certain rickettsial organisms. However, it is not seen in epidemic typhus (*Rickettsia prowazekii*) or murine typhus (*R. typhi*) and is rarely observed in Rocky Mountain spotted fever (*R. rickettsii*). African tick-bite fever and the similar Mediterranean tick-bite fever (*R. conorii*) are usually mild and self-limiting infections, occasionally associated with a rash and fever with lymphadenopathy. Symptomatic illnesses can be shortened with doxycycline.

Cutaneous anthrax occurs after *Bacillus anthracis* spores are inoculated through skin abrasions or via biting flies. After a short incubation period of 2–5 days a papule forms which becomes vesicular. Patients have fever with malaise and local adenopathy. The surrounding oedema is often prominent and can lead to airway compromise with neck lesions. The vesicle ruptures and forms a black eschar 1 week later. Although very rare in the UK, sporadic cases can occur (vets, farmers, abattoir workers). The use of 'weaponised' anthrax spores by terrorists (as found in letters to US senators in 2001) unfortunately remains a possibility in the future, therefore such a lesion in certain patients, including Post Office staff, should raise alarm bells.

The characteristic lesion of bubonic plague is the bubo, a painful, suppurating lymph node mass, usually in the groin or axilla; it is associated with severe constitutional symptoms. An important differential diagnosis of bubonic plague (and anthrax) is ulceroglandular tularaemia (*Francisella tularensis*). These two organisms are also favourites of biological weapon researchers and may pose a risk in the future.

The characteristic rash of Lyme disease is erythema chronicum migrans (see also *Book 1* – Cardiology Question 8). This rash begins as a papule at the site of an infected tick bite after 1–20 days. It then expands with central clearing and a raised erythematous edge. From this edge *Borrelia burgdorferi* can be isolated.

Case 32

1 **D** Intravenous (iv) broad-spectrum antibiotics
  E Transfer to high dependency unit
  F Aggressive fluid resuscitation

2 **D** He should receive meningococcal group C vaccination.

This young, asplenic man has septic shock, probably caused by *Streptococcus pneumoniae*. He needs to be transferred to a high dependency unit.

The spleen can be thought of as a sieve that removes microbes and blood cells from the circulation. The remaining reticuloendothelial system can partially compensate for its absence but cannot adequately remove encapsulated bacteria and intracellular parasites from the bloodstream. Patients are therefore at greatly increased risk of sepsis and overwhelming infection due to *S. pneumoniae, Haemophilus influenzae* type B, and *Neisseria meningitidis,* and are at increased risk of severe parasitic infections such as malaria, babesiosis, and ehrlichiosis. Other bacterial causes of post-splenectomy sepsis include *Salmonella* spp., *Pseudomonas aeruginosa*, enterobacteriaceae, group B streptococci, and *Capnocytophaga canimorsis* (from dog and cat bites).

Post-splenectomy sepsis (PSS) is most common within the first 2 years after the operation and in children. Patients usually develop a short 'flu-like' illness over 1–2 days, which is followed by an abrupt and profound deterioration. This can result in fulminant infection, termed overwhelming post-splenectomy infection (OPSI).

PSS traditionally had a mortality of >50% despite appropriate treatment (although this may now be 10–20%), two-thirds of deaths occurring within the first 24-h of presentation. The risks of PSS and OPSI can be reduced if clinical guidelines are followed.[8] Important points include:

- Patients should be vaccinated at least 2 weeks before an elective splenectomy or at 2 weeks following an emergency operation. Pneumococcal, Hib, and meningococcal group C vaccinations are recommended. Annual influenza immunisation should also be offered. The unconjugated pneumococcal vaccine is currently recommended, although the newer conjugate vaccine may have a future role. A booster should be given at 5-yearly intervals.
- Patients require lifelong daily penicillin V or erythromycin as prophylaxis.
- The patient should carry a letter or wear a bracelet or pendant alerting medical staff to their splenectomy.
- Patient education – they need to present to hospital if symptomatic and understand the risks of foreign travel to take appropriate precautions.
- Urgent use of broad-spectrum antibiotics if PSS is suspected. Empiric therapy would include an extended spectrum cephalosporin or carbapenem plus vancomycin plus a flouroquinolone.

Post-splenectomy infection patients are not at increased risk of cytomegalovirus (CMV) or *Pneumocystis jiroveci* (*P. carinii*) infection.

Case 33

1   E   *Haemophilus influenzae* B vaccination.

This lady has CSF rhinorrhoea following a basal skull fracture. NB – a diagnostic test would be to send the fluid to biochemistry: CSF contains glucose but mucus does not.

Although these patients are at an increased risk of bacterial meningitis, prophylactic antibiotics, eg daily penicillin V, have not been shown to reduce its incidence. However, meningococcal (A and C), pneumococcal, and Hib vaccinations have been shown to be of benefit and should be given.

Although some leaks resolve spontaneously, others are amenable to, or require, neurosurgical intervention. Cadaveric grafts are no longer used because of the possibility of transmitting Creutzfeld Jacob disease. A blood patch is used to help post LP head and back ache.

Case 34

1 **E** Herpes simplex encephalitis

2 **D** CSF PCR

See answer to Chapter 2, Case 3, pages 109–111.

A sagittal venous thrombosis is associated with severe headache, altered consciousness and localising signs. It is associated with: anti-phospholipid syndrome, Factor V Leiden deficiency, thrombocythaemia, polycythaemia, Behcet's disease, nephrotic syndrome and the combined oral contraceptive pill.

Case 35

1 **A** MRI spine

2 **B** Bone marrow culture

Brucellosis is a systemic disease caused by bacteria from the *Brucella* genus, which has naturally occurring reservoirs in animals. Four species are known to be pathogenic in humans with *Brucella melitensis* being the most virulent:

- *Brucella melitensis* – goats, sheep, camels
- *Brucella abortus* – cattle, buffalo, camels, yaks
- *Brucella suis* –pigs
- *Brucella canis* – dogs.
- *Brucella* sp. are Gram-negative intracellular coccobacilli.

There are no specific symptoms or classic signs for brucellosis and the condition can present acutely or more indolently. The more frequent associations are listed below:

- Fever
- Constitutional symptoms – fatigue, malaise, anorexia
- Musculoskeletal symptoms – low back pain, spine and joint tenderness
- GI symptoms – abdominal pain, diarrhoea or constipation, hepatomegaly, splenomegaly.

Eating or drinking unpasteurised goat's milk and related dairy products is the main route of transmission of *Brucella melitensis* to humans.

Investigation of brucellosis:

- FBC – leukopenia or pancytopenia
- LFT – transaminitis

- Blood cultures – *B. melitensis* and *B. suis* are the more likely to have bacteraemia. The likelihood of successful culture decreases for all strains as the disease duration progresses
- *Brucella*-specific serology – positive when titres ≥1 : 160 or when a four-fold rise in titre is demonstrated in convalescent sera
- Bone marrow cultures are typically more sensitive than blood cultures. Culture is often positive in the absence of positive blood cultures and serological results
- Histology – granuloma formation is seen, especially on liver biopsy
- Imaging
  X-ray –AP lumbar spinal and sacroiliac X-ray – sacroiliitis
  MRI – best to identify degree of vertebral involvement, risk of vertebral collapse and to exclude abscess formation

Treatment of brucellosis is always with combination antibiotic therapy

- Doxycycline + rifampacin
- Doxycycline + an aminoglycoside
- If complications develop (see below) then prolonged courses of the above are given.

Complications of brucellosis:

- Bone and joint lesions
- Infective endocarditis
- CNS involvement – meningitis or encephalitis

Case 36

1   **D**   Tuberculosis

2   **A**   Colonoscopy plus biopsy

Abdominal tuberculosis occurs in approximately 2% of patients with TB and is more frequent in patients with HIV co-infection. The most common site involved is the ileocaecal junction, possibly as a result of increased physiological stasis, increased rate of fluid and electrolyte absorption, minimal digestive activity and the large proportion of lymphoid tissue. Other sites can include the omentum, liver, spleen and peritoneum and can result in clinical ascites, adhesion formation, hepatosplenomegaly and bowel obstruction. Diarrhoea is the result of ileocaecal obstruction that leads to a proximal bacterial overgrowth.

The onset of disease is usually insidious with symptoms present for several months before diagnosis. The most common presentations are:

- Colicky abdominal pain, vomiting and abdominal distension
- Insidious onset of abdominal distension and ascites (peritoneal involvement)
- Incidental and asymptomatic.

Colonoscopy is less invasive compared to an ultrasound-guided biopsy, especially in the presence of ascites because it helps to reduce the risk of bacterial peritonitis and of sepsis, persistent leakage of ascites, and haematoma formation. Colonoscopy is useful to assess mucosal lesions involving the terminal ileum, caecum and throughout the colon, and to allow for accurate biopsies – especially as the differential diagnosis would include an ileocaecal tumour.

Staining ascitic fluid for AFB is infrequently positive and culture takes up to 8 weeks and even then may be negative. If it was an option – laparoscopy is the gold standard test for diagnosing intra-abdominal TB, where the tuberculous lesions can be directly visualised in the peritoneum.

CA-125 is not a specific tumour marker for ovarian cancer. Serum CA-125 is elevated in several other physiological and pathological conditions. CA-125 antigen is also found on both healthy and malignant cells of mesothelial tissue (pleura, pericardium, peritoneum, endometrium). Hence any condition causing ascites can cause a raised CA-125 level.

- Malignant causes:
     Ovarian cancer
     Endometrial cancer
     Pancreatic cancer
     Colon cancer
- Non-malignant:
     Pregnancy
     Endometriosis
     Salpingitis
     Chronic liver disease
     Chronic renal failure
     Acute pancreatitis
     Abdominal TB.

Case 37

1   C   ITU referral, intubation, central-line insertion, iv quinine, haemofiltration

This patient has severe cerebral malaria due to *Plasmodium falciparum*. In endemic areas it is easy to contract malaria in cities as well as in rural parts.

The World Health Organization definition of cerebral malaria requires:

- Unarousable coma
- Evidence of acute infection with *P. falciparum*
- No other identifiable cause of coma.

Steroids are not recommended in cerebral malaria

Indicators of severity of *P. falciparum*: (*see Chapter 2, Case 4*)

The treatment of cerebral malaria entails:

- Chloroquine resistance is frequently seen in most areas where malaria is endemic, and so iv quinine is the drug of choice
- Intubation is indicated with a GCS <8/15
- Renal failure in severe malaria is common and can require haemofiltration
- Seek specialist advice in a complicated cases

Case 38

1   B   Send isolate to Reference Laboratory

Multi-drug-resistant tuberculosis (MDRTB) is TB that is isolated and resistant to isoniazid and rifampicin. There are two types of MDRTB:

- Acquired MDRTB – following inadequate previous TB treatment in an individual
- Initial MDRTB – where the index case is transmitting MDR infection; this reflects poor TB control programmes in a community over time.

TB is the second most common infectious disease in terms of adult mortality, causing approximately two million deaths a year worldwide. WHO estimates that one-third of the world's population is infected with *Mycobacterium tuberculosis*.

The World Heath Organization and International Union Against Tuberculosis and Lung Disease (WHO/IUATLD) Global Project on Drug Resistance Surveillance has found MDRTB (prevalence >4% among new TB cases) in Eastern Europe (Estonia, Latvia), Latin America (Argentina), Africa and Asia. With the rapid increase in globalisation, trans-national migration and tourism, all countries are potential targets for outbreaks of MDRTB.

While fully sensitive TB can be cured within 6 months, forms of drug-resistant TB require extensive chemotherapy for up to 2 years with agents that carry greater risks of side-effects:

- Spectinomycin
- Ofloxacin.

Rapid conformation of resistance can be confirmed by PCR for mutations in the *RpoB* gene, associated with rifampicin resistance, a marker of multi-drug resistance.

Spot urine testing will help to assess adherence to therapy with the presence of red-coloured urine, but will not aid in the assessment of treatment success.

Case 39

1   E   Leptospirosis

The patient has leptospirosis – caused by the spirochaete *Leptospira interrogans* – this is a common zoonotic infection worldwide. Synonyms such as swamp fever, cane-cutter fever, swineherd's disease, rice-field fever, mud fever, Stuttgart disease, and Canicola are from where attempts have been made to link specific serovars with specific animals, geographical areas or behaviour – mostly erroneously – and are best avoided.

The natural hosts for *L. interrogans* are mammals and man is only incidentally infected, usually by contact with infected urine – usually in contaminated freshwater or soil. *L. interrogans* is classified into various serovars some of which have distinct animal hosts including rats (*L. interrogans* serovar Icterohaemorrhagiae), dogs (serovar Canicola), as well as cats and livestock. Leptospires nest in the tubules of mammalian kidneys and are excreted in the urine. They can survive for several months in warm (> 22°C) and a neutral pH (6.2–8.0); these conditions occur all year round in the tropics but only in summer and autumn in temperate climes. The organism enters the body through abrasions in the skin or the mucosal surfaces of the eye, mouth, nasopharynx or oesophagus.

The epidemiology has changed in recent years and the risk factors for leptospirosis are best considered in this order – certainly in the West:

1. Recreational – canoeing, windsurfing, swimming, waterskiing, white-water rafting and fishing – especially if lakes or reservoirs have contact with contaminated animal urine.

2. Domestic – handling animals at home, rainwater collecting systems.

3. Occupational – livestock farmers, milking workers, vets, plumbers, sewerage workers, abattoir workers, coal miners and those in the fishing industry.

While infection with leptospira is most often asymptomatic or so mild as to be ignored, in diagnosed cases the incubation period is a median of 10 days with a range of 2–26 days – the duration of which has no significance; the clinical features include:

- A self limiting illness (in 90%) consisting of
    abrupt onset of fever (often >40°C) and rigors

myalgia, often excruciating – of the thighs, calves, back and abdomen

abdominal pain together with wall tenderness can mimic an acute abdomen

nausea, vomiting, diarrhoea and a sore throat are common symptoms

headache

cough and chest pain can occur

examination may reveal

> conjunctival suffusion – easily overlooked and a useful diagnostic clue. Pus and serous secretions are absent and there is no matting of the eyelashes and eyelids
>
> less useful and more vague signs include:
>> pharyngeal injection
>> rash
>> hepatomegaly and/or mild splenomegaly
>> lymphadenopathy

Leptospira may be found in the blood, CSF and tissues

after 4–7 days improvement may occur from this 'bacteraemic' phase

- After 2–5 days patients can deteriorate with milder and more variable symptoms. Leptospira disappear from the blood and appear in the urine, the antibody titre rises, hence the 'immune' phase. The features are:

  fever

  worsening headache and meningism (>50%) – the hallmark of this phase

- The biphasic description above is often overstated and not at all a classic feature of icteric leptospirosis/ Weil's disease

- Icteric leptospirosis/ Weil's disease – 10% of leptospirosis

  alongside the above features, in this dramatic variant (particularly associated with the more virulent serovars eg serovar Ictrohaemorrhagiae) one sees jaundice, renal dysfunction, myocarditis, haemorrhagic manifestations and a high mortality rate (>10%)

  icterus occurs about the 5th to 9th day and remains for about a month; its presence or absence (not depth) is critical – virtually all deaths from Weil's disease occur in icteric cases, however the deaths do not occur from liver failure

  hepatomegaly with percussion tenderness is a good marker of disease activity

  conjunctival haemorrhage is an extremely useful diagnostic sign, especially together with icterus and conjunctival suffusion

  purpura, petechiae, bleeding of the gums, mild haemoptysis occur

  death may occur from sub-arachnoid haemorrhage or exsanguination from the GI tract renal failure can occur rapidly, oliguria or anuria usually develops in the second week (maybe earlier). Presentation with anuria does occur and is a grave sign as it is usually too late to affect the natural history of the disease

disturbance of consciousness is usually due to uraemic encephalopathy in these cases, cf. aseptic meningitis in mild early cases

Diagnosis

- Neutrophilia is usual; anaemia occurs frequently and is multifactorial – blood loss, azotaemia and haemolysis contribute; thrombocytopaenia occurs in severe cases in a consumptive coagulopathy, fragments would be expected on a film (DIC)
- Urinalysis shows proteinuria, pyuria and microscopic haematuria
- U&E – renal failure and sometimes hypokalaemia (renal loss)
- Hyperbilirubinaemia (conjugated predominates), elevated ALP and transaminitis (from hepatic necrosis, but greater than five-fold increases are exceptional)
- CK – elevated from skeletal muscle damage in the first week of the illness
- PT prolongation (easily corrected with vitamin K)
- CXR – show a variety of abnormalities, none is pathognomic, most commonly one sees small, patchy, peripheral, snow-flake alveolar shadowing corresponding to alveolar haemorrhage in severe cases

Definitive diagnosis

- Blood and CSF culture during the first week or urine culture in the second week are possible, but technically difficult and the lab must know leptospirosis is being considered so special media can be used. Culture results are not known for 4–6 weeks and as such are no use to the severely unwell hospitalised patient
- Serology is most useful
    microscopic agglutination test (MAT) is the reference standard but technically difficult
        most specific when a four fold difference between acute and convalescent titres is seen
        antibody titre ≥ 1:100 with symptoms is suggestive
    IgM ELISA or CFT are commercially available, performed at 7–14 days they compare well to MAT; if positive, samples can then be sent on to the reference lab for MAT

Treatment

- Mild disease – many recover without treatment within 10–14 days, otherwise doxycycline, ampicillin or amoxicillin are useful and can shorted the duration of the illness

- Severe disease – parenteral penicillin G or erythromycin alongside full supportive care of the affected organs – kidneys, liver, lungs and CNS.

Case 40

1   A   Acute CMV infection

Fever in a patient following solid organ transplantation has a wide differential diagnosis because of the confounding iatrogenic immunosuppression.

Infection	Time scale of presentation post transplant
Bacterial urine infection	1–2 weeks
Clostridium difficile	1–2 weeks (post antibiotics)
Aspergillus infection	2–6 weeks
CMV infection	4-12 weeks
Parvovirus B19 infection	4–12 weeks
Cryptosporidium parvum	4–24 weeks

Acute CMV infection is related to the CMV status of the donor and the degree of immunosuppression. Donor–recipient CMV antibody status matching is desirable. If the recipient was CMV negative and the donor was CMV IgG positive then the risk of acute CMV in the recipient is high. CMV infection can also be transmitted through transfused blood products. Leukopenia is suggestive of CMV infection.

Symptoms relate to the site of infection:

- GI tract – diarrhoea, abdominal pain
- Chest – pneumonitis
- CNS – encephalitis, retinitis
- Abdomen – hepatitis.

Parvovirus B19 results in an isolated anaemia – although this could be the result of the immunosuppressant agents used.

A baseline CMV serology and PCR result help to assess for risk, and a repeat CMV PCR at the time of presentation can speed up diagnosis.

Treatment of acute CMV infection:

Four antiviral agents have activity against CMV (cf *Chapter 1, Case 6 page 98*)

- Ganciclovir iv – first-line therapy
- Valganciclovir oral
- Foscarnet iv – used rarely because markedly nephrotoxic
- Cidofovir iv – used rarely because markedly nephrotoxic.

Case 41

1   **A**   Acute typhoid fever

See answer to Chapter 2, Case 10 pages 102 and 103.

Case 42

1   **C**   Splenic aspirate

Visceral leishmaniasis (VL) is usually caused by species from the genus *Leishmania* usually – as is likely in this case – *Leishmania donovani* (*L. donovani donovani, L. donovani chagasi or L. donovani infantum; L. braziliensis* complex is occasionally involved), which is transmitted by the bite of the female sandfly. Ninety percent of new cases in the world arise in rural areas of the Indian subcontinent, Afghanistan, Nepal, Bangladesh, Brazil and East Africa, but it has a worldwide distribution being endemic in southern Europe for example. Blood borne transmission between iv drug users is common, with many infections occurring in HIV infected patients.

In this case the travel history (Kenya and Sudan), fever, splenomegaly and leukopaenia all suggest VL. The differential diagnosis would also include:

• Malaria
• TB
• Enteric fever
• Tropical splenomegaly syndrome
• Schistosomiasis

Following an incubation period of 2–12 months the following features develop insidiously:

• Fever – continuous or intermittent
• Weight loss
• Night sweats
• Abdominal discomfort
• Diarrhoea
• Hepatomegaly
• Splenomegaly – moderate or massive
• Lymphadenopathy
• Darkening of the skin – hence the name 'kala-azar', black fever

Investigations

• FBC – anaemia, leukopaenia or pancytopaenia
• The diagnosis is made by demonstrating amastigotes (Leishman-Donovan bodies)

bone marrow aspirate is the most satisfactory technique (*qv Book 3 – Haematology Question 8*)

Giemsa stained bone marrow smears may reveal the amastigotes

culture is possible on NNN media and takes one to three weeks splenic aspirate and culture has the highest yield but has more complications

liver and lymph nodes can also be biopsied

- Serology – detects antibody to K39 antigen of *L. donovani* by ELISA or IFAT
- Speciation can be performed by PCR of tissue or a culture specimen

Treatment

- Liposomal amphotericin B iv – is the most useful treatment in the developed world
- Sodium stibogluconate iv or im (painful) – a pentavalent antimonial is an alternative in the developing world
- Miltefosine – an oral agent, has promise for the future

In HIV the response to treatment is slower, require longer treatment and are more likely to relapse

Without treatment VL has a mortality of over 90%.

Complications include haemorrhage, severe anaemia and secondary bacterial infection.

Case 43

1   D   Erythromycin

This patient has an atypical pneumonia due to *Mycoplasma pneumoniae*.

Mycoplasma pneumoniae is a common cause of atypical pneumonia and most commonly affects people aged less than 40. Various studies suggest that it causes 15–50% of all pneumonia in adults and an even higher percentage of pneumonia in school-aged children.

People at highest risk for mycoplasma pneumonia include those living or working in crowded areas such as schools and homeless shelters, although many people who contract mycoplasma pneumonia have no identifiable risk factor.

Clinical features:

- Headache
- Fever and rigors
- Cough – often non-productive
- Sore throat.

Less frequent symptoms include:

- Skin lesions – erythema multiforme, erythema nodosum
- Arthralgia.

Causes of erythema multiforme:

- Infections – herpes simplex, *Mycoplasma pneumoniae*
- Drugs – sulphonamides, penicillins, tetracyclines, phenytoin
- Vaccinations
- Vasculitic disorders – Wegener's granulomatosis
- Idiopathic.

Diagnosis:

- Sputum culture – it is a slow-growing organism
- CXR – diffuse reticulonodular or interstitial infiltrates affecting the lower lobes, 20% have a pleural effusion, lobar consolidation is uncommon
- Serology – a four-fold rise in complement fixation test (CFT) antibody titres between acute-phase and convalescent-phase serum specimens, ideally obtained 2–3 weeks apart.

Treatment:

- Macrolide antibiotics are most effective – erythromycin, clarithromycin, azithromycin
- Oral steroids are a treatment for autoimmune-related erythema multiforme – but not for that with an infective cause.
- Ciprofloxacin is not routinely used for treatment of mycoplasma pneumonia although the newer quinolones (ofloxacin) are under review.

Complications:

- Meningoencephalitis
- Guillain–Barré syndrome
- Transverse myelitis
- Myopericarditis
- Cardiac arrhythmias
- Raynaud's phenomenon
- Haemolytic anaemia
- Disseminated intravascular coagulation.

See Book 1, Chapter 2 (Respiratory Medicine), Case 2.

Case 44

1   E   Cryoglobulins

This gentleman presents with fever, ankle oedema, hypertension, proteinuria, microscopic haematuria, anaemia and renal failure. Clinically he has acute nephritic syndrome resulting from cryoglobulinaemia due to chronic hepatitis C infection.

HIV-associated nephropathy (HIV-AN) is characterised by proteinuria, renal impairment, normal 'bright' kidneys on ultrasound, normal blood pressure and focal segmental glomerulosclerosis (FSGS) on renal biopsy (cf *Book 2* – Renal medicine Case 2 p. 125).

Tests for the cause of the acute nephritic syndrome include:

- Throat swab culture – post-streptococcal GN
- Serum complement (C3 and C4) – immune complex GN, post-infective GN, cryglobulinaemia
- ANCA – Wegener's granulomatosis, microscopic polyangiitis, Churg–Strauss syndrome
- Anti-glomerular basement membrane antibody (GBM) – Goodpasture's syndrome.

Chronic hepatitis C infection is associated with a number of extra-hepatic conditions:

- Essential mixed cryoglobulinaemia
- Porphyria cutanea tarda
- Membranoproliferative glomerulonephritis
- Lichen planus (cf *Book 2* – Dermatology Case 12 p 14)
- B-cell non-Hodgkin's lymphoma.

Case 45

1   D   *Legionella pneumophila*

2   C   Clarithromycin

Legionella pneumophilia is an obligate Gram-negative bacillus.

The classical presentation begins with an incubation period of 2–10 days.

Patients often experience a prodrome of 1–2 days of mild headache and myalgias, followed by high fever, chills, and multiple rigors.

- Cough – present in 90%, is usually non-productive initially but may become productive
- Other chest symptoms – dyspnoea, pleuritic chest pain, and haemoptysis

- GI symptoms – nausea, vomiting, diarrhoea
- CNS symptoms – headache, altered mental status, and rarely, focal neurology
- Musculoskeletal symptoms – arthralgia and myalgia.

Transmission of legionella bacteria is through aerosols from infected water sources:

- Cooling systems
- Showers
- Decorative fountains
- Humidifiers
- Respiratory therapy equipment
- Whirlpool spas.

Investigation of Legionnaires' disease:

- FBC – leukocytosis
- U&E – watch for hyponatraemia as a consequence of SIADH or with renal impairment as a result of acute GN
- LFT – hyperbilirubinaemia, transaminitis or elevated ALP
- CK – can be raised because of rhabdomyolysis
- Urine dipstick – proteinuria, haematuria
- Sputum and blood cultures – *Legionella pneumophila* isolation
- ABG – hypoxia
- Serology
  Urine antigen testing is highly specific, sensitive, and very rapid, or
  Use direct fluorescent antibody testing
- CXR – 50% have pleural effusion.

Treatment of Legionnaires' disease:

- Macrolides – clarithromycin, erythromycin, or azithromycin

(cf *Book 1* – Respiratory Questions 1 and 8)

Case 46

1   **D**   *Streptococcus viridans*

This woman clinically has infective endocarditis.

Organism	Frequency of cases isolated
Streptococcus viridans	50%
Staphylococcus aureus	20%
Enterococcus sp	10%

Other organisms less frequently isolated include:

- Gram-negative bacilli
- HACEK organisms – *Haemophilus* sp, *Actinobacillus* sp, *Cardiobacterium* sp, *Eikenella* sp, *Kingella* sp.
- *Staphylococcus epidermidis* – more common post valve replacement, along with *S. aureus*
- *Coxiella burnetii* is the causative agent for Q fever – Q fever endocarditis usually complicates chronic Q fever in the presence of a prosthetic valve.

(cf *Chapter 2, Case 21, pages 133 and 134*)

(cf *Book 1* – Cardiology questions 27, 29, 31)

Case 47

1   A   Itraconazole

This woman has acute pulmonary histoplasmosis following exposure and infection with the fungus *Histoplasma capsulatum* that is predominantly found in river valleys in North and Central America. It is the commonest cause of fungal lung disease; the pathogen is found in soil, particularly near bat and bird habitats and is spread by inhalation. The incubation period is 5–18 days.

- Over 90% of patients are asymptomatic. The clinical features of infection are:
- Acute pulmonary histoplasmosis – one sees dyspnoea, cough and chest pain. If severe, sweats, fever, malaise, myalgia and weight loss occur
- A rheumatological syndrome of erythema multiforme, arthritis and erythema nodosum occurs in 5–6 %
- Chronic disease develops after the illness or years later. One sees chronic pulmonary histoplasmosis and chronic disseminated histoplasmosis involving the reticuloendothelial system and adrenal glands (Addison's can occur as long as 30 years after leaving the endemic area), hepatosplenomegaly may rarely be seen. This is the most recognised pattern of disease outside endemic areas.
- There is considerable variation in the rate of progression of acute histoplasmosis that has spread beyond the lung. At the extremes of age and in the immunocompromised it can be particularly rapid with infiltration of the reticuloendothelial system, liver, spleen and bone marrow; purpura and bleeding from thrombocytopaenia can occur and even pancytopaenia, meningo-encephalitis is unusual as is superior vena caval obstruction

Diagnosis of acute pulmonary histoplasmosis

- CXR – is often normal, but the most common finding is hilar and mediastinal lymphadenopathy. In severe cases diffuse reticulonodular shadowing is seen. Cavitation is rare
- Microscopy and culture of sputum or biopsy samples – culture on Sabouraud's medium
- Serology – CFT – titre ≥1:32 equates to active infection
- Blood culture is rarely positive in acute disease

The acute disease is usually self-limiting so treatment is unnecessary. If treatment is necessary consider and azole eg itraconazole or ketoconazole

Chronic disease requires treatment with liposomal amphotericin B followed by prolonged treatment with itraconazole. New agents such as posaconazole are likely to have a future role. Steroids are not indicated.

Complications:

- Pericarditis
- Cardiac tamponade

Case 48

1   **D**   Genotype 2

Non-adjustable factors

- Viral genotype – the major viral factor which determines the likelihood of achieving a sustained viral response following a complete course of antiviral therapy for hepatitis C. Patients with genotypes 2 and 3 are almost three times more likely than patients with genotype 1 to respond to therapy.
- Viral load – in immunosuppressed individuals the viral load can be very high – HIV co-infection or post liver transplant. In these circumstances, the high viral titre combined with poor tolerance to antiviral therapy for hepatitis C reduces the likelihood of an SVR.
- Degree of hepatic fibrosis – published data show that the greater the degree of hepatic fibrosis the lower the response to antiviral therapy. Combining ribavirin with PEG-IFN has improved the chance of SVR to just over 40%, but this figure falls short of what can be achieved in individuals without cirrhosis.

Adjustable factors

- Alcohol consumption – retrospective data show that alcohol consumption both before and during treatment may influence the outcome of therapy, above and beyond the effects of alcohol in causing more rapid disease progression and influencing adherence. It is recommended that patients abstain from alcohol before and during antiviral therapy for hepatitis C.

- Age – the likelihood of achieving SVR diminishes by about 5% per decade so it has been suggested that individuals with non-favourable genotypes are treated earlier to maximise the chance for SVR.

REFERENCES

1. Costabel, U., Guzman, J. 2001. Bronchoalveolar lavage in interstitial lung disease. *Current Opinions in Pulmonary Medicine* 7(5), 255–61.
2. http://www.gmc-uk.org/guidance/library/serious_communicable_diseases.asp
3. Maskell, N.A., Butland, R.J.A. 2003. BTS guidelines for the investigation of a unilateral pleural effusion in adults. *Thorax* 58(Suppl. II), ii8–ii17.
4. Davies, C.W.H. *et al.* 2003. BTS guidelines for the management of pleural infection. *Thorax* 58(Suppl. II), ii18–ii28.
5. Bernard, G.R., Vincent, J.L. *et al.* Recombinant human protein C Worldwide Evaluation in Severe Sepsis (PROWESS) study group. 2001. Related Articles, Links Efficacy and safety of recombinant human activated protein C for severe sepsis. *New England Journal of Medicine* 344(10), 699–709. Pubmed ID: 11236773.
6. Department of Health website: www.immunisation.nhs.uk
7. *Health Information for Overseas Travellers* (the 'yellow book') and *Immunisation against Infectious Disease* (the 'green book') can be found at http://www.dh.gov.uk
8. Davies, J.M., Barnes, R., Milligan, D. 2002. Update of guidelines for the prevention and treatment of infection in patients with an absent or dysfunctional spleen. *Clinical Medicine* 2(5), 440–3.

INDEX

Locators in normal type refer to the Questions section, locators in **bold** type refer to the Answers section.